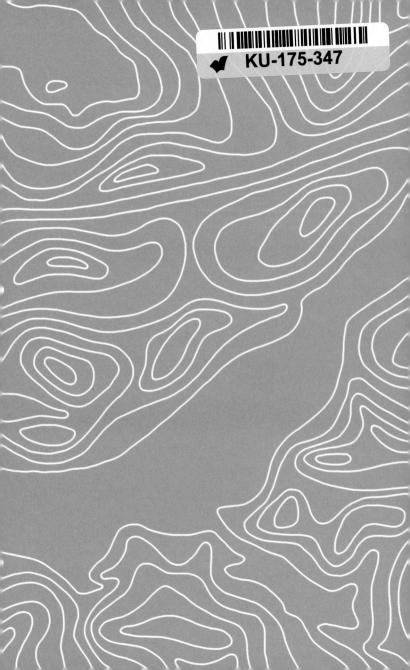

Libby DeLana

Do Walk

Navigate earth, mind and body.
Step by step.

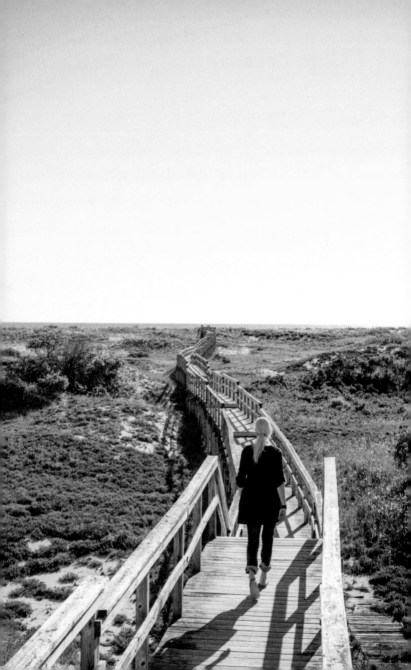

An illuminating book that powerfully conveys a simple truth: that putting one foot in front of the other is a transformative act. DeLana writes with insight, heart and wit about love, loss, work, creativity and the mysteries of being human. *Do Walk* is a moving and wise book about one woman's long path toward enlightenment, that also tells a story about all of us.

Cheryl Strayed

For William and Orren.
You are wonderful.

Published by
The Do Book Company 2021
Works in Progress Publishing Ltd
thedobook.co

Text and photography
© Libby DeLana 2021
p4 © Michael Piazza
p28 © Dom Francis Pellegrino
p109 © Chris Dempsey

The right of Libby DeLana to be
identified as author of this work has
been asserted by her in accordance
with the Copyright, Designs and
Patents Act 1988

To find out more about our company,
books and authors, please visit
thedobook.co or follow us **@dobookco**

5 per cent of our proceeds from the sale
of this book is given to The Do Lectures
to help it achieve its aim of making
positive change: **thedolectures.com**

Cover designed by James Victore
Book designed and set by Ratiotype
Endpaper design based on contour
map of Newburyport, MA

Printed and bound by OZGraf Print
on Munken, an FSC-certified paper

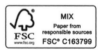

MIX
Paper from
responsible sources
FSC® C163799

A CIP catalogue record for this book
is available from the British Library

ISBN 978-1-907974-96-0

10 9 8 7 6 5 4 3 2 1

Contents

Prologue   10

Introduction   14

1. This morning walk   20

2. Every damn day   28

3. Feet on the ground, eyes to the sky   42

4. The alchemy of sensing   50

5. A creative practice   64

6. Finding momentum   72

7. Fresh-air medicine   82

8. A way of being   90

9. Keep going   98

Walking mantra   111

FAQ   113

Resources   120

About the Author   123

Thanks   124

All walking is discovery.
On foot, we take the time
to see things whole.

Hal Borland

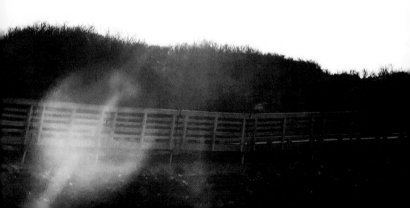

We walk for all kinds of reasons: to get groceries, go into town, travel to a friend's house, walk a dog, clear our heads or find inspiration. They all have value.

My MorningWalk — I refer to my daily practice of walking as 'MorningWalk' throughout this book — can be all that and something more. It has become a meditative practice, and therefore a bit different from simply 'going for a walk'. As with seated meditation, this practice mirrors the realities of life, the details of each day, changing and moving constantly. MorningWalk embraces connection, observation, movement and constant change. It has become my paradigm for a way of being in the world, in harmony with the way the natural world operates.

Walking is rather narrowly understood, but it has the potential to be life changing. To understand it as life changing requires a clarity of intention, surrender of destination, dedication to the moment, and commitment to a practice. Your MorningWalk may not look like my MorningWalk, and that is wonderful. It may be in an urban neighbourhood or a rural community; it may include wheels; it may include a furry companion, or not. No matter where or how you go, there you are: committed to a practice, open to the moment and embracing the ever-changing circumstances.

Come, join me on a MorningWalk.

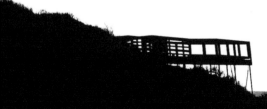

Prologue

It is 5:02 am, a Tuesday morning in September 2020; the cool air is beginning to replace the slow, humid, heavy air of summer. It is noticeably darker at this time in the morning than it was a week ago. I must admit there is a lovely anticipation of the coming autumn months but also a hint of dread as the deep cold of a New England winter is just weeks away. Changing seasons make the world feel hopeful, familiar and promising. They are a powerful reminder that change is the natural state of affairs. These inevitable shifts can bring with them a beautiful feeling of newness and also the feeling that nothing is stable. Walking in every distinct and unique season has been a series of glorious and unyielding lessons. An ongoing lesson in transformation, in embracing all that is in each unique moment.

Every morning when I pull on my shoes and head out the door, I am inspired by how walking every damn day has fundamentally changed my life. There are the obvious shifts in fitness level, increased appetite, better sleep and more perspective, but the subtle shifts are perhaps where the magic resides. My sense of time has changed. My understanding of distance has forever been re-modelled. Step by singular step, I have walked over 25,000 miles, enough miles to circumnavigate the earth. This has taken me nine years. I no longer think of this as 'just a morning walk'. I now call it 'my MorningWalk', a sacred act to start the day. This, however, wasn't always the case.

When I first committed to going for a walk every day, I had to get over my athletic ego. I had spent much of my life defined as 'an athlete'. During my high-school years I played field hockey, basketball and lacrosse and, by my senior year, I was captain of all three teams. In college I started rowing, and did that for four years, including competing in the National Championships. For decades, my self-worth came from how well I played. So, when I started to … walk … it took me, in truth, a year or two to get comfortable with something so low key. I would eventually come to understand that MorningWalk wasn't an athletic endeavour: it was something else.

Looking back, I can see that MorningWalk has been a serendipitous pilgrimage of sorts. A surprising journey, a daily adventure: cold, hot, sunny, rainy, boring, exciting, joyous, heavy, creative, innovative, and loving. When I started I didn't know the profound impact it would have on my life. In fact, at the time it felt like a small gesture, a simple dedication of some time to get outside and go for a walk. After nine years of walking every day it has become an essential practice that feels like devotion — perhaps even prayer.

The important thing has not been the mileage or how fast; in fact, I am very aware that many have run / walked / biked / hiked / rolled 25,000+ miles in a much shorter time frame, or perhaps have had a similar practice for many more years than I. If you are an avid runner then undoubtedly you have already covered these miles over the course of your life. I have friends and colleagues who I think of as The Original Walkers; I think some of them have had a MorningWalk practice for several decades and likely have walked the distance to the moon and back. No, MorningWalk isn't about how many miles or how many years — although those are markers of a sort — instead it is about the loyalty and enthusiasm for each walk. It became a subtle practice that saved me. It saved my spirit. It saved my way of being. Ultimately, it reminded me who I am.

This isn't a book about walking as an act of redemption — it is about a slow, natural realisation that there is great joy that can come from a wildly simple change and commitment in your life. MorningWalk is a micro daily habit that has the potential of having a macro lifelong impact. It is a gentle, slow practice ... and pace (not speed) matters. There is no rushing, no urgency embedded into a step. It isn't a task to 'get over' so I can move on to the next thing on the list. Instead it is an opportunity to be aligned with the pace of the natural world. I had lost touch with that. My days had become 'to do' lists and looking at the clock to get to the next thing on time.

In fact, when I look to the natural world the only things that move quickly, with urgency and speed, are things that are often destructive: nor'easters, earthquakes, hurricanes, wildfires. Life was moving too quickly. There was too much untethered energy. Walking was a way back to a pace that was natural and recognisable, and also a way to truly be open, to see what each day was going to bring. Mama Nature has her own pace and the 21st-century world has a different energy and pace that felt out of alignment to me. The 'normal' societal pace meant that I had forgotten we are part of the natural world, with a need to slow down before we can really understand, know and hear what we need.

MorningWalk has become a way of life. It is a subtle, cumulative, spiritual, physical, creative, healing, unhurried, essential practice that has required discipline, commitment and a splash of wild optimism to make it profoundly impactful. Walking is what makes us human.

To go for a walk is perhaps one of the most primal things we do each day. A dear friend, Eric, when asked how he was, would always answer: 'I'm fine. I am walking the earth.' Walking the earth has been a way to ground myself, to center myself, to find the heartbeat both in myself and of a place, a road, a path, a walkway, a sidewalk, a field .... This book is a thanksgiving for MorningWalk.

Walk as if you are kissing the Earth with your feet.

Thich Nhat Hanh

Introduction

So, what exactly is MorningWalk? Why does it matter? And why the morning rather than a lovely wind-down at the end of the day? Well, here is the thing: the most generous act we can make is to take time to focus on our own wellbeing as soon as we wake up (in most cases, that is the morning). There is something about a morning ritual that creates a sense of comfort, of certainty, of hope, or contentment.

The invitation is to place your attention on the sensation of your foot touching the ground as you wake up, a practice to cultivate awareness around balance and energy. MorningWalk is a daily moving meditation much like yoga or qigong. It requires a slowing down of thought. Step by step. Breath by breath. Tenderly. Thoughtfully. Without an agenda. Without a goal. A way to start the day with focus on the present moment. For me it is a gesture that says, 'Welcome to right now.' The Greek physician Hippocrates (c. 460–370BC) famously claimed that 'walking is the best medicine'. I would have to agree.

Humans need to move. We are built for it. Our days in the 21st century are often filled to the brim with sitting indoors, in cars, unmoving. Walking stimulates not only the body but also the mind. Creativity, innovation, focus, wonder; these are just some of our companions when we walk.

But why the morning? To kick off your day on the right foot. Once you commit that time to yourself there is a certain private satisfaction and personal fulfilment that comes from starting the day with a focus on your wellbeing. There is scientific evidence indicating that early risers tend to be quite proactive and happier. As Laura Garnett points out in a 2020 article for *Inc*: 'increased productivity isn't the only bonus to getting up early, you'll also be happier. According to a University of Toronto study, morning people reported higher levels of happiness.' MorningWalk has made that wholeheartedly true for me.

I have never regretted going for a walk, even though there are certainly some walks that have been unpleasant. It could be the weather. It could be a state of mind. It could be what happened the day before. It could be remembering that thing I said, that I wish I hadn't. All the things that are prickly or troublesome have to have their time. I have found that the best way to manage or navigate those emotions is by adding a bit of motion to them. Movement prevents the challenging times from getting stuck in my body.

Sometimes a walk can be challenging. This morning, for instance, I went for a walk in a gale-force wind with local flooding and a temperature of 6°C (42°F). I wore the wrong clothes. About 20 minutes into the walk I was completely wet from head to toe, so wet that I found myself wringing out my mittens every 15 minutes because they were waterlogged. While, yes, there was a certain element of this MorningWalk that was terribly uncomfortable, verging on too cold, I was with two friends who found the whole situation wonderfully entertaining. We were warm 'enough' and we knew that we'd be home within an hour or so to hot tea and dry clothes. Life lesson learned: We can do hard stuff and hard stuff is temporary.

I do not want to suggest that going on a MorningWalk without the proper gear, precautions, nourishment and safety measures is a viable way to 'learn lessons'. We need to start with safety. Please be sure that someone—a friend, family member, neighbour, housemate or colleague—knows where you will be. I put in my coat pockets a little laminated card with emergency contacts and make sure that is all updated on my phone. Be sure to have the proper gear, shoes, hat, warm clothes, water, snack, sunscreen, headlamp, reflective gear, etc. (more on that in Chapter 2). And lastly, please carry with you some type of safety device. I have my phone and I now carry a whistle with me. There are also some handy little devices that can fit into your pocket that will flash a strobe light and sound an alarm. Consider something like that. Fortunately, I've never had to use any of these things.

OK, safety briefing over. Who's ready to venture out?

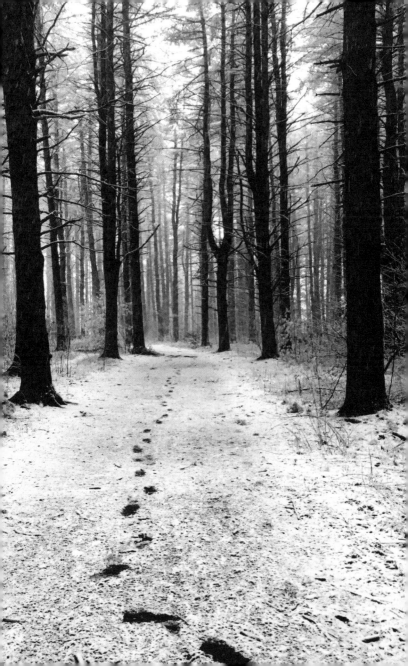

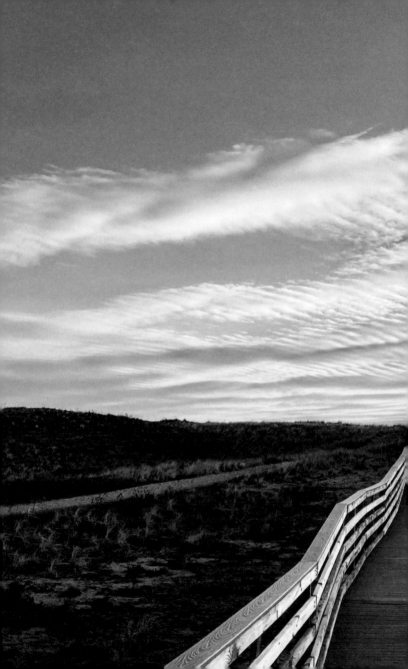

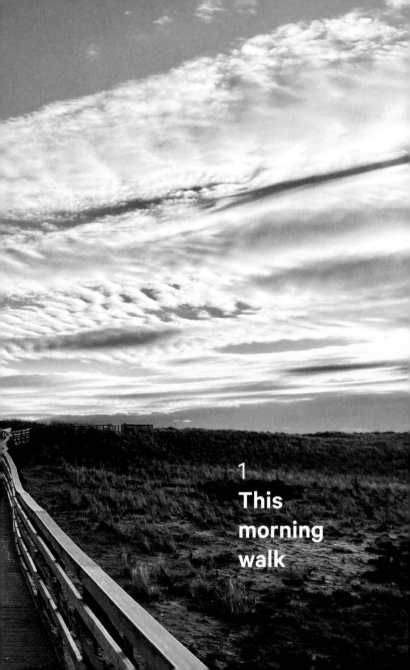

1
This
morning
walk

What a glorious morning. Cold, bright, hopeful, and feeling grateful. I started this practice because I needed to get back to a bigger sense of purpose and clarity, one that began with a fundamental intimacy with the earth. On this morning, I have seen the sun come up, a coyote, several blue jays, an eagle, and the start to my 54th year. I have come to realise that making a commitment and following through with it is what love looks like. This hasn't been an easy path these last five years or so, but I haven't missed a day. Some walks have felt impossible. Yet every walk has been a gift. An opportunity to add energy, focus and space to the day. Space to hold overwhelming thoughts, to hear essential intuition, to toss around silly ideas, to look at gut reactions, to play with messy concepts, to feel grateful and to celebrate another pass around the sun. Happy birthday to me.

I had no idea the impact a simple, gentle walk would have on my life. The impact comes not only from the actual physical walking but also from the discipline, the practice, the commitment. This MorningWalk has ignited my sense of curiosity, satiated my everlasting wanderlust and been the most powerful tool for inspiration in my life.

I walk roughly the same loop most days. Out the front door, 5am, 8.2 miles, 17,740 steps. I walk past the same barn. On the same path. Along the same river. With the same headwind around that last turn. This conscious repetition is a form of meditation, designed for intentional familiarity. It's almost as if I could do this route blindfolded, I have travelled it so often. Some days, on the backstretch, I close my eyes while walking for 10, 20, 30, 40 steps. This creates a powerful silence. In this silence, I can hear what my body — my gut, my heart — is telling me in this moment. The mindlessness of the route itself brings mindfulness to the moment.

It seems so obvious now but my initial intention was simple: to be outside and to be mindful. Every day. To create space. To find time for creativity. To dedicate an hour of my day to something nourishing and satisfying. As my days had become more about tasks to complete, it became increasingly obvious that I needed to get outdoors, move and play a little.

This is not a story about mileage or pace. In fact, it is the opposite. This is a story about listening, seeing, hearing, feeling and understanding. It is also a story of radical self-care. At the start, I wouldn't have been able to identify it that way, but as time has passed the discipline of doing something physically and emotionally nourishing every day has been the most profound outcome of this daily practice.

Redefining success

When I think about life before the covid pandemic of 2020–2021, it felt as if the world defined success as someone who was busy. The cult of busy was overwhelming. MorningWalk became an act of rebellion that challenged the cultural norm. Success became more about going out even when it was −28°C (−18°F), when it was pouring with rain, when I 'didn't have time' or when I just plain old didn't want to go. Success was going because I'd promised myself I would, not because anyone else noticed or cared. It was a wildly selfish pursuit. I was able to redefine success in terms that were profoundly simple — to have walked every day — and to recognise that there wasn't one walk where I didn't feel better. And what do I mean by 'feel better'? Well, everything. As it turns out, persistence, focus and determination can stretch limits and push boundaries. That is a powerful feeling of freedom and love. Commitment is intoxicating. There is nothing more generous than sticking to a promise you have made to yourself.

**I only went out for a walk and finally
concluded to stay out till sundown,
for going out, I found, was really going in.**

John Muir

I dare say that is why pilgrims, protestors, monks, hikers,
wanderers, activists, explorers, adventurers and poets often
walk. There is a freedom when we walk. We strip away all
the unnecessary noise and details in our mind and in the
world and step into a place of profound sense of agency
and focused attention. This is my experience with the ritual
of a MorningWalk. Silence and celebration. Freedom and
love. Quiet, intimate, daily acknowledgements of strength,
commitment and resilience. This is why I feel better after
a walk. It is a personal triumph.

There are many other benefits of a good walk. Walking
is said to provide some powerful health benefits, such as:

— Improves circulation
— Strengthens bones
— Improves sleep
— Boosts energy for the day
— Maintains weight / burns calories
— Improves mood
— Strengthens your heart
— Boosts immune function
— Can help lower blood sugar
— Supports joints
— Lowers Alzheimer risks

One morning, late in the autumn of 2011, I struggled to get out of bed. I hadn't slept well. I wanted to stay put. I hadn't been doing my MorningWalk for long, but had come to know that walking was my best bet. There is always something that happens on a MorningWalk that improves the upcoming day. I've since learned that the days I don't want to go are in fact the days I most 'need' to go.

The morning before, I thought I had seen two coyotes at the end of the street. So, driven by curiosity, not commitment or joy, I meandered downstairs to get my gear on and headed out the door. It was just after 5am and was pitch-black out, with a cold sliver of a moon and a cloud layer that made it feel as if there was no light in the world. I waited until I got to the end of the street before I turned on my headlamp, because there is something about gently, very gently, easing into the silent darkness of a walk. By keeping my headlamp off it felt as if I was quietly entering the morning. The stillness of the dark felt like a hug. It's interesting, there is a quiet, determined community up at this hour. I saw a familiar runner at the top of the street. We all recognise each other but don't really know anything about one another. We nod and wave, it feels like a secret handshake when our paths cross.

Later, after passing my familiar morning squad, I saw the quick-moving shadow of something larger than a dog … It was the coyote. The discreet nature of how this animal exists in the world is fascinating. It made me pause. Humans are so loud, so dominant, so obvious. We exist in our ecosystems flamboyantly and overtly. The coyote, however, is intimately integrated into its private world. Quietly powerful, discreet in its movement and impact. There were lessons to be learned from this morning visitor. My MorningWalk offers up many a teacher. I was glad curiosity got the better of me that morning.

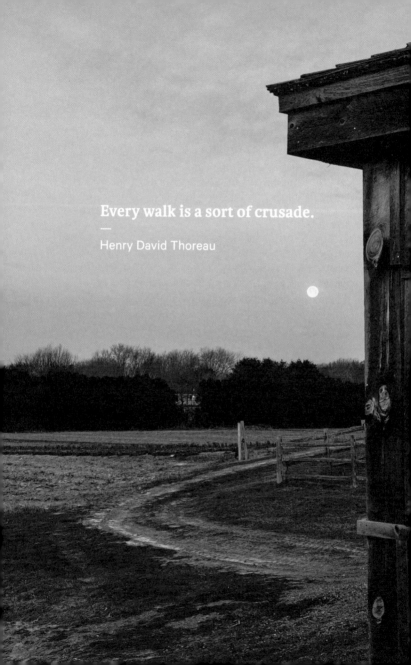

Every walk is a sort of crusade.

—

Henry David Thoreau

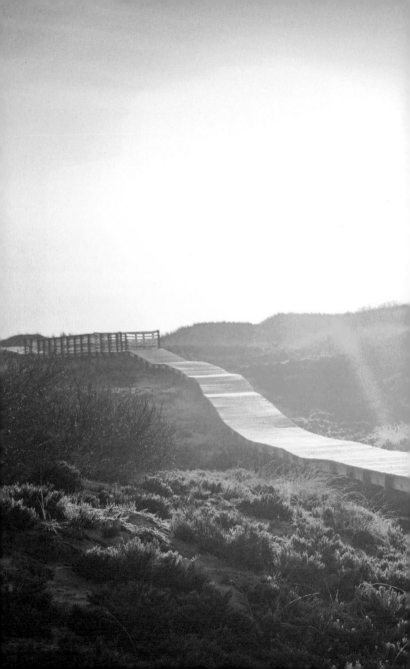

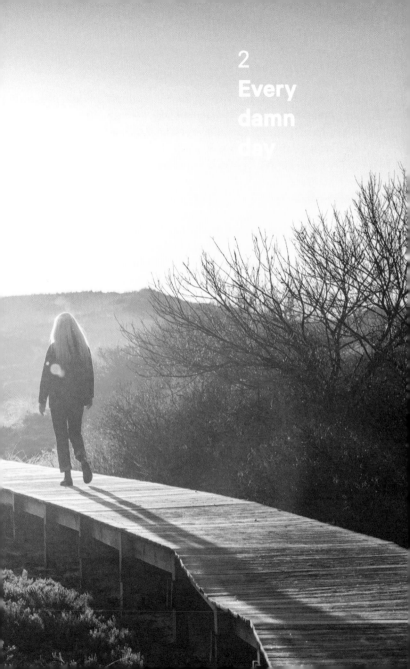

2
**Every
damn
day**

It feels as if the sun has been up for hours when I get out the door. It is 5am, and already hot with the humidity of the day. Humidity makes everything feel slow. Very slow. I don't seem to have the pep in my walking. Today it feels heavy. Yet there is a reverie to the slowness, to the stillness. I feel as if I see everything unfolding, blooming. All of the roses, daisies, ferns, dogwood trees and lavender are just days away from their full glory. My deliberately slower pace today helps me see that. The other reason I can see this unfurling and blossoming is because I go every day. I have the previous day, the previous week, to measure against. At this time last week, the roses were still in bud; today, I not only see the pink-tinged petals sprinkled with gold dust but also smell the lemony, deliciously crisp fragrance. These roses are truly enchanting. Here is the beauty of doing something daily: it enables us to see clearly, know deeply, and understand our world more intimately.

Small rituals can be a joyous way to kickstart the day and at the same time provide powerful comfort. A walk, a cup of tea, breath work, making the bed, morning pages. I knew a daily ritual had the potential to be a tool to engage my mind, a way to clear the trash out of my head, a daily dose of beauty and physical satisfaction, an ongoing source of humility and a generous wellspring of contentment in the certainty of it; but I didn't realise until years into this practice how essential it would become.

Having grown up as an athlete, I understood the power of a daily practice, the ritual of coming together to work towards a common goal and the dedication to action. Much of my time in high school was spent on a playing field or court. I loved the repetition, the physicality, the competition, the community, the team, the dose of dopamine. It was the 1980s and girls with muscles and a fierce sense of competition and commitment to daily action were not accepted by the norms of the culture back then. In our high school, we dressed for practice in the girls' bathroom, which was not large enough for all of us. We didn't have a changing room as the boys did, but no matter — in some ways, it made us stronger. What I realised at that formative time in life was that a daily physical practice, as part of a community, was essential. I also learned that holding true to the bravery required to do the things society insisted that you shouldn't or couldn't do was profoundly satisfying. These lessons, learned in my teens but perhaps not fully realised then, have informed my daily practice of walking — to walk every single day, with a faithfulness to action and a commitment to learning.

MorningWalk is essential for many reasons: it starts the day off right, builds momentum and gives structure to the day. It helps me recognise the power of prioritising, builds confidence, reminds me that success comes step by step, and ensures I do something well. Back in school, those daily practices were formational in the way I lived my day. Each day I had a certain amount of energy to spend — my energy bank. I had to be thoughtful about how I would spend this currency, what I was going to focus on, what gave me more strength during the day. I found consistently that after practice each day I would have *more* energy, *more* focus and *more* momentum. Doing something you love, even physical activity, generates more energy rather than depleting it.

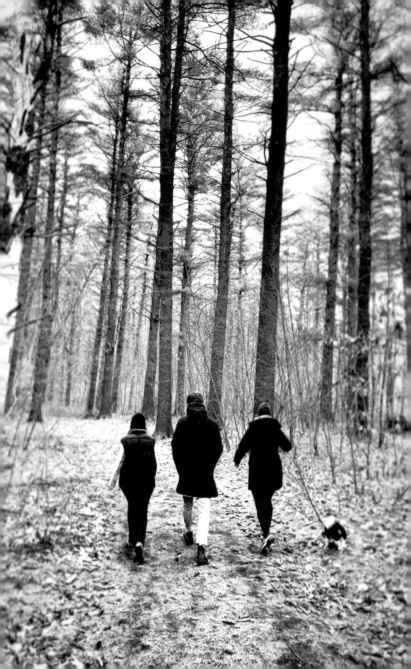

Here are a few things to consider when building a daily walking practice:

TIP 1 — Find a point of motivation
Ask yourself why you are adding this to your life. Self-care? Exercise? A time to recharge? A place to problem-solve or create? You may need to remind yourself on the more challenging days.

TIP 2 — Start simply
Start with something doable in terms of time and distance. Ask yourself: How much time can I commit over the course of the next month? Can I carve out 15, 20, 30 minutes each day? This will help determine your route. A walk around the neighbourhood is a wonderful way to begin. Start small; take the first steps. Repeat for 5 days. Repeat again.

TIP 3 — Stick to it for a month, without fail
It takes three to four weeks for something to become essential, for something to become a habit.

TIP 4 — Do it without judgement, just walk
Try it. See how you feel. I decided initially to commit to every damn day, because for me it was helpful to not give myself an out: too cold, too rainy, too tired. But that might not work for you, and that's OK. The pace doesn't matter, the distance doesn't matter. Just walk.

TIP 5 — Prepare thoughtfully
Set a wake-up time. Get your things ready the night before. Ask yourself, what will help me get from waking to walking? Is there one thing that feels like a barrier — cold toes and hands? How can I eliminate that barrier? For me it was double socks and toe warmers.

TIP 6 — Keep a routine

It takes a splash of perseverance to make a habit stick, so honouring the routine — same time, same place — will help build your walking practice. 'Once it's a habit, exercise feels easier and doesn't take as much willpower when you don't feel like it,' says Charles Duhigg, author of *The Power of Habit.*

TIP 7 — Invite others to join you

Having a walking partner can be a wonderful way to keep you motivated — that sense of someone counting on you can help get you out of bed. (Also, for me, during the covid pandemic walking became a vital source of community.) Ask yourself, who might be willing to join me? Even if it isn't every day.

TIP 8 — Acknowledge the time

Accept that you may have to give something up to create the time and space for this new practice. I believe we don't just *find* time for things that matter — we *make* time. Ask yourself, what am I willing to do (or stop doing) to make this happen?

TIP 9 — Record your walks

Keep track of your walks. Ask yourself, how can I build in a bit of accountability and record-keeping so that when I look back I am reminded of the walk? Make a note, tell a friend, take a picture. Note how you feel at the end of each walk. A walk brings its own lessons, challenges and rewards. I have never been on a walk where I didn't feel better after. Never. Keep track and enjoy looking back.

TIP 10 — Observe the times when it isn't fun

There is a lot to learn from the hard walks. Ask yourself, what on earth was that? What just happened? What was hard about it? What did I take away from it?

Hard walks. Oh yes, the hard, long, cold, wet, snowy, icy, dark walks. It is often in the hard walks where I find the most information. December 2017, it was 0°c (32°F) and according to the weather app I use it would 'feel like −19°c (12°F)' because of the angry wind whipping off the Atlantic Ocean from the north-east. Around here that is called a nor'easter. Nor'easters are often violent storms where Mama Nature growls and shows her teeth. It is clear that on these mornings the lesson becomes very simple: slow down, stay warm, take it step by step, stay very alert to this moment.

On this morning, it literally was step by icy step. Each time I put my foot down it would slide out. The earth was not stable. This walk felt chaotic and uncertain. As I came to the end of Hay Street about to turn on to Green my feet came out from under me and I crashed down and spilled all over the place, ending up with my ass squarely on the ice and my hat and mittens somewhere over there. It was basically a yard sale. It's a long way down for me, as I am six feet tall. After the initial surprise of the moment and checking to see if anything hurt, I had to laugh. I had become distracted by something inconsequential. I had lost track of each step just for a moment. I wasn't present. I laughed because there was clearly a larger lesson in that walk. That moment. Stay present.

The basics

Let's talk gear. What does it take to get started and walk regularly? Well, one of the wonderful things about walking is there isn't much you need to purchase. A good pair of walking boots or running shoes is the only essential element. Take care of your feet. An investment in good shoes has a long-term impact on your wellbeing. What else you need may depend on where in the world you'll be walking and how changeable the weather is, but here's what I use.

My everyday essentials:

— **Running shoes** (changed out every 600 miles). When I get a new pair of shoes I put the date on the insole to make sure I swap them out appropriately. If possible, go to a running shop, try on several brands and have the experts help you find the right shoe. If you don't have access to a running shop then why not ask a friend who is a runner what they use? Having ill-fitting shoes is the most common reason for injury. Consider the tread and the surfaces you will be travelling the most on: sidewalks, woodland paths, ice.

— **Wool socks.** Find a well-fitting sock to prevent blisters. I love 'old man' wool socks, not 'performance' socks. When it's cold I wear two pairs.

— **Sports bra.** The right size will make you much more comfortable. Have a few so you can rotate, and they'll last longer if you don't put them in the tumble dryer.

— **Joggers or leggings.** Look for technical fabrics as they will hold up a lot better with regular washing. I have a few pairs: one pair for the winter that are fleece-lined, a lighter pair for summer, and a magical pair with a pocket for when I find the perfect pine cone.

— **Technical-fabric long-sleeved T-shirt.** I wear long sleeves, for both sun protection and a comforting layer.

— **Running belt.** I use this to carry my phone if I'm not wearing a layer with pockets.

- **Headlamp**
- **Reflective leg bands**
- **Dog-deterrent spray** (that I have never used)
- **Fitness tracker**
- **Phone or whistle**

Below zero (32°F):

- **Toe warmers** (shoe inserts)
- **Fleece leggings over tights**
- **Wool long-sleeved shirt**
- **Heavy technical-fabric top with thumbholes**
- **Down vest**
- **Down jacket**
- **Fleece neck gaiter** (you could use a snood or a scarf)
- **Warm hat**
- **Gloves or mittens, reflective**

I've included a fitness tracker on my list, although that is not necessary. Initially I used one simply because I was curious. As I've already said, the intention of MorningWalk is not how many steps, how far, how fast or how long. But you might find it interesting to know the scope of your route.

Preparing to walk

An important thing would be to check in with your doctor about any injuries or health conditions that may need to be considered before starting a regular MorningWalk practice. I have over the last few years developed some sore spots and various little aches and pains, but nothing truly of note.

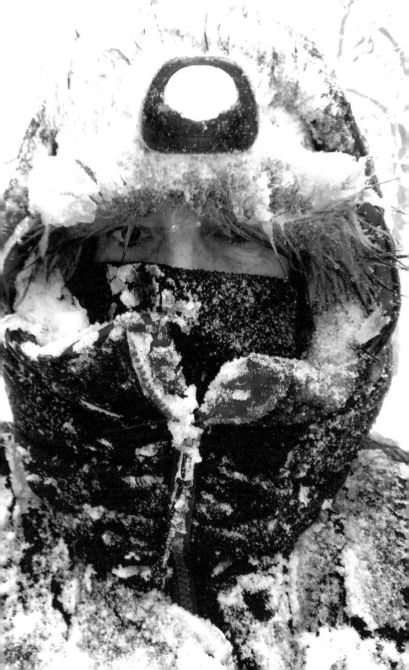

That, in fact, is one of the great things about walking. We are built to do it. There are very few ways to get injured while walking. I feel it is something I/we can do forever.

That being said, there are a few things you can do to prevent the most common injuries.

— Be sure to stay hydrated throughout your walk and your day

— Do some simple leg stretches before heading out the door

— And if anything begins to hurt consistently, please stop and seek the advice of a doctor

I am often asked if I listen to anything while I walk. Podcasts? Music? Books? The answer is yes to all of those but not every day. I find that on the days I walk without any distraction I am more attentive to the moment, the world. And there are some days when I am listening to something as a means of distraction. Maybe there is something I don't want to acknowledge, think about or tend to, so I pop in the earphones. Sometimes I don't even realise I've done that until I'm back home. I'll have walked 10 miles and not really remembered much of it. It is on those days that I might go out for another walk later in the day to tune in, get grounded and address what is happening.

I do find, however, there are some audiobooks that are made for walking; travel stories that are an antidote for wanderlust. They transport you to another place even though you have merely stepped out the back door. This can be a wonderful adventure for those of us with virtually insatiable adventurous spirit.

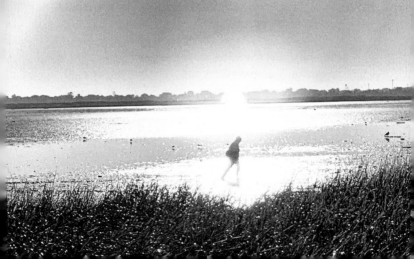

The journey of a thousand miles begins with one step.

—

Lao Tzu

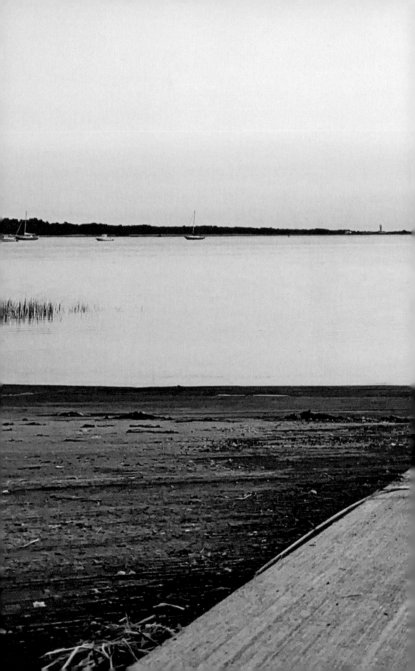

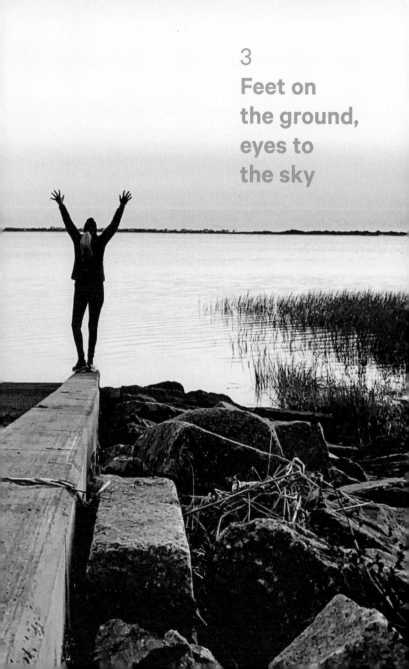

3
Feet on the ground, eyes to the sky

I can't seem to find my way. I am trying to navigate through downtown Los Angeles, a city I am not very familiar with, and it feels a bit overwhelming. Not scary, just uncertain. I have to be at a meeting in an hour and I'm not sure you can get anywhere in LA in an hour, especially by foot. Despite my good sense of direction, of which I am absurdly proud, I can't seem to navigate my way out of this one neighbourhood. I literally feel as if I am walking around and around, despite the GPS on my phone telling me where to go. It is so frustrating and the anxiety of being late for this new business meeting feels sucky.

Then I remember. Stop. Get grounded and look up. I literally stop on the sidewalk, step off to the side, put my phone down and focus on finding my feet, on getting grounded. What do I mean by 'finding my feet'? It feels something like being on a rollercoaster, then coming to a stop and actually noticing where you are. It is becoming aware of the specifics of your place and location.

I pause and stop, then look up. There is something about looking at the treetops, the rooflines, where the sun is in the sky and, in this case, the mountain range to the north, that creates signposts to help me navigate beyond the street names and intersections. I begin walking again and get to the meeting on time.

Get grounded. Look up. Walk forward. Step by step.

The truth of the matter is there are many 'ways' and 'reasons' to walk. Walk for health, walk for fitness, walk for connection, walk for clarity, walk for grounding, walk to get from point A to point B. MorningWalk embodies all of that and is about staying connected to the world, and to the present moment. Much like in meditation or yoga, attention brought to our bodies and our breath has a profound impact. Inevitably, each MorningWalk has a pace and tenor of its own, and is a reflection of that day, that moment, that mood.

MorningWalk is a great barometer for what is happening in your world both internally and externally at any given time. A MorningWalk that feels slow and laboured may reflect the internal energy of what is happening in your thoughts. A brisk walk is often an indicator of excitement about an idea or a newfound energy your body feels at that moment. Once we connect to where we are with our thoughts and our body, we are able to get curious and learn. Because the act of walking doesn't require much critical attention, we can use the rhythm and momentum to focus on things happening right now. MorningWalk has the potential to center our thoughts. When I notice that my thoughts are off somewhere else, I often say to myself, 'Welcome to right now.'

Of course, there are some days when I get home and realise I have barely noticed a thing on my walk. Was it foggy? Did I move quickly or slowly? Did I hear the birds or notice the sunrise? No. My mind was racing the whole time. I was playing out scenarios that hadn't even happened yet. Trying to solve problems that didn't exist. I was so preoccupied with 'what ifs' that I didn't notice what was happening in the moment. Life was simply passing by without recognition. My attention was not connected to now or here. I was not at all grounded.

Staying grounded adds magic to any day. It is where distraction meets intention and focus. If we spend our walks thinking about this afternoon, tonight and tomorrow, the beauty and opportunity of right now disappear. When I am walking, all the clues to solving issues are at hand, but if I am not listening or attentive to those clues I miss key information. Attention is essential. When you have things on your mind, as we all do, walking helps to sort the mind. *Solvitur ambulando* is a Latin phrase that means 'it is solved by walking'.

It is now well understood that walking outdoors in nature can have a significant impact on both physical and mental health. An emerging practice of walking barefoot, or 'earthing', has begun to be recognised for its healing power. Earthing is simple: connect your feet or hands directly to the earth. Literally, find a clean, safe patch of sand, grass, even concrete, and take off your shoes.

I must admit when I first heard about earthing I was uncertain and curious about the impact. I cast my mind back to days in childhood spent barefoot, and how delicious that was. I was certainly willing to try it out, so for the past few months I have picked a day to go for a quick walk barefoot. It is getting increasingly difficult as winter rolls in, however my understanding is that winter is a powerful time to do it regardless of the cold — but briefly and carefully.

> **We can see the cold not as an adversarial, malignant, or negative power, but instead as a mirror that reflects whether or not our body is responding the right way, the way nature intended.**
>
> Wim Hof

There is some interesting research about the concept of earthing, also called grounding, which suggest that the connection between humans and the earth's subtle electric charge has been lost due to such aspects of modern life as insulated buildings and footwear. As Carrie Dennett explains in the *Washington Post*: 'Advocates of grounding say this disconnect might be contributing to the chronic diseases that are particularly prevalent in industrialised societies. … Research has shown barefoot contact with the earth can produce nearly instant changes in a variety of physiological measures, helping improve sleep, reduce pain, decrease muscle tension and lower stress.' And what's more, it's free and available without a prescription!

'Feet on the ground, eyes to the sky' has become a kind of mantra or intention on many of my walks. It is a reminder to embrace where you are at any given moment. There is a combination of optimism and reality that feels just right. And, during the covid pandemic, both were required: optimism and reality. Recently I have taken walks with friends while they remain in their apartment building, simply walking around the space that is available. We call each other and 'walk' wherever we are, together.

Regardless of where you live, it is possible to add more walking to your day. Remember, a MorningWalk can be a few blocks with several deep breaths embedded into it. If you happen to live in a location that means you spend a great deal of time in the car, consider parking at the far end of the car park. And if you get to a building where there is a choice of walking up a flight of stairs or using a lift, take the stairs. We can all fit more walking into our day regardless of where we live.

Harvard Health reported recently: 'A study of 12,000 adults found that people who live in cities have a lower risk of being overweight and obese than people who live in the suburbs. In Atlanta, for example, 45 per cent of suburban men were overweight and 23 per cent were obese; among urbanites, however, only 37 per cent were overweight and 13 per cent obese.' The explanation? Driving vs walking. People in cities walk more. There is a website called WalkScore that enables you to find the walkability rating of a place. I use it when travelling and find it to be a wonderful tool to get to know a location prior to arrival.

I had a friend who once said that jet lag was the spirit trying to catch up with the physical movement of the body flying from one place to another. Walking is an antidote to the wild speed at which we live our lives, to our insistence on rushing and doing everything quickly. It allows us to exist at a similar pace to our natural environment, even when we are in an urban setting. When I arrive in a new place the first thing I do is get on my walking shoes and slowly begin to acquaint myself with where I am, to help piece together the neighbourhoods and landscapes. In this moment there is no destination, only a desire to get acquainted and grounded.

Walking is a practice of being tuned into one's body. So now that we are grounded, let's tune into the senses.

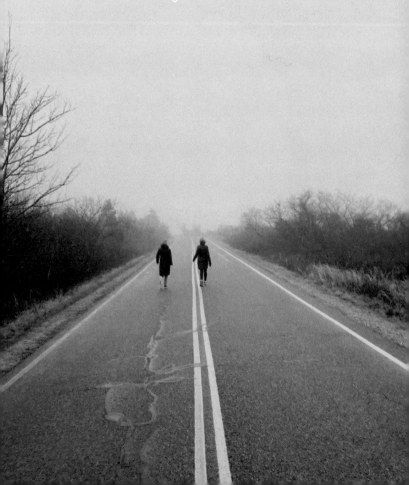

If one just keeps on walking,
everything will be all right.
—

Søren Kierkegaard

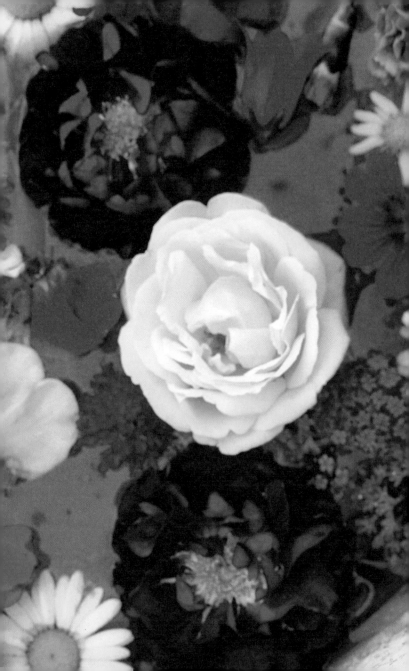

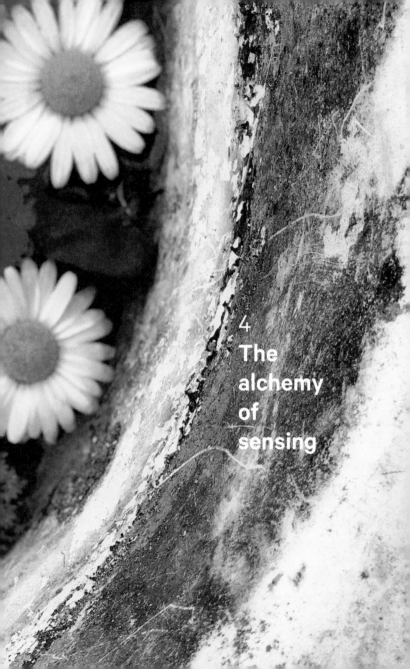

4
The alchemy of sensing

It is beginning to warm up in the northeast, which means fewer layers. This is a welcome relief. There are some April days it is so cold that it takes 20 minutes to get all the layers on and get the gear together before I head out the door.

But not today, and it made walking feel a little more relaxed and brighter. I wasn't bracing against the cold, making sure to cover all exposed skin. I could enjoy the moment more fully rather than endure it. Walking in the middle of the winter has its own pleasures, but it's nothing compared to the sun coming up a bit earlier and feeling the warmth on my face. Interestingly, because I am not focused on keeping warm or staying upright on the black ice, I am able to see and hear more. All my senses kick into high gear.

Today, the air smelled like those precious few days when the ocean makes itself known: briney and alive. The morning smelled like the taste of salt itself. The wind on my cheeks felt hopeful rather than angry and the chorus of birds' elation for the coming spring was effervescent. That being said, there was so much trash in my head that I found it hard to host these good feelings. Unsettled, I needed to walk more than usual. Today it took 12 miles.

It is interesting to watch my mind while walking. On this day, I was so consumed by my thinking that it was impossible to acknowledge anything else. I almost talked myself out of going at all. 'You should rest.' 'Take a day off.' I pulled on my shoes and opened the door. 'Good job, get walking. Remember, there has never been a walk where you didn't feel better at the end.' ... 'Slow down. Pause. Feel that warm breeze on your cheeks.' ... 'Ahhhhh, now close your eyes and take a deep breath in. Smell the Atlantic Ocean. Hear the bird song.'

With each step, the heaviness in my thinking began to lighten. The senses came online and the message was simple: you are part of a larger ecosystem. Tap into it. Our thoughts are just that, simply thoughts. We can tell ourselves all sorts of stories but sometimes what we really need to do is pause and recognise that there is a whole wide world out here, waiting for us to notice. Walking with presence is a reminder to see, hear, smell and feel the world. With each step the trash in my head is recycled and left at the curb.

On the days when my head isn't full of junky thoughts, the opportunity to harness the power of each step for problem-solving is tremendous. Understand and clarify an issue, step by step. Consider possible solutions, step by step. Develop a plan, step by step. There are days when I feel as if I have solved all of the world's problems and created the next most important thing for humanity, while walking. MorningWalk has never been boring, despite the many miles. It is such a powerful tool for expanding thinking. As Albert Einstein said, 'It's not that I'm so smart, it's just that I stay with problems longer.' To dedicate time to a subject, to allow for deep thinking and to use all of our senses in that process: this is the way we get to true creativity and perhaps invention.

I was in advertising for 30 years and once had a creative director who would say: 'Throw away the first five thoughts, because the true, unique and original thinking only comes after you dismiss the obvious.' MorningWalk allows for this kind of deep work. Original thoughts require play, innovation requires experimentation, and walking creates the necessary space and momentum. MorningWalk provides a constant source of inspiration when you can open up to all of your senses.

> **If you seek creative ideas go walking. Angels whisper to a man when he goes for a walk.**
>
> —
>
> Raymond I. Myers

I must admit that for years I didn't pay attention. I missed things. I overlooked, ignored and didn't recognise the opportunity to bring a brighter awareness to all the senses while walking. When I realised what I was missing, it made me think of my bulletin board at work.

In my office, I used to have an enormous bulletin board next to my desk with images on it from various sources:

photos from trips, pages of magazines, illustrators' work, tear sheets from photographers, a beautiful little red cashmere thread, a little bundle of leaves from a glorious hike, a handwritten note from a friend, a printout of a passage from one of my favourite books. This board served as a testing ground, an idea farm, a place where things could collide visually to generate a new idea. A MorningWalk has the same elements. The added benefit of a walk is the opportunity to pull information from every one of the senses, not just the visual. Every walk I see something new, hear something different, even when I am doing the exact same walk as the previous day. The unique shade of each sunrise is a palette I have rarely seen before and it sparks a new way of thinking about colour. Geese overhead and crashing waves inspire an entirely new soundtrack.

Listen

I once worked with an amazing musician who, when he ran, tested and sketched new songs with each step. The tempo of a passing train on the tracks sounded like a high hat which, mixed with the horns from the motorbikes zooming past, created a baseline for him to work from. He would record his voice with the orchestra of the city behind him as he ran. MorningWalk has the potential to provide the creative alchemy we need. I often think of him when I pull on my sparkle boots in the morning and set out into my own world of inspiration.

See

Recently I was walking past our local farm. In the front of the farm shop they have an old Victorian bathtub, rusted on the outside and bright white on the inside. This day the tub was filled with clear water and dozens of flowers: dahlias, chamomile, lavender, zinnias. It was a riot of colour, texture and proportion. As I approached, I had to stop. There was a solution in that tub to something I was working on: a luxury wild skincare line. Much like the bulletin board in my office, this too was a place for unexpected juxtapositions that unlocked a new idea. I plunged my hands into the water, smelled the lavender, looked closely into the faces of the dahlias and zinnias — and there I found the colours for this new brand.

I no longer look, I see. Most of our life we look at something but don't fully take it in. Truly seeing something requires a pace at which you can appreciate its entirety, even the things that may not be visible at first glance. Think of the sunrise that subtly changes colour each second. Or a hummingbird that one minute looks draped in a silvery dress and the next is wearing a green jacket. Ephemeral beauty.

A friend once said something funny to me that reinforced my appreciation for the pace of walking. 'You never see people running through art galleries.' Fair point. *Looking* is a gesture. It is the taking in of information, while *seeing* allows for the entity to be understood. This happens at walking pace.

Smell

Walks have a fragrance. Have you ever been out and about and smelled wood smoke, cookies baking, or a pine tree? What about an orange blossom or a still lake? These fragrances instantly transport you back to a time and place when perhaps you first experienced it. Scents are powerful. And evocative. Scents tell a story or provoke a vibrant memory. One reason is that the olfactory system

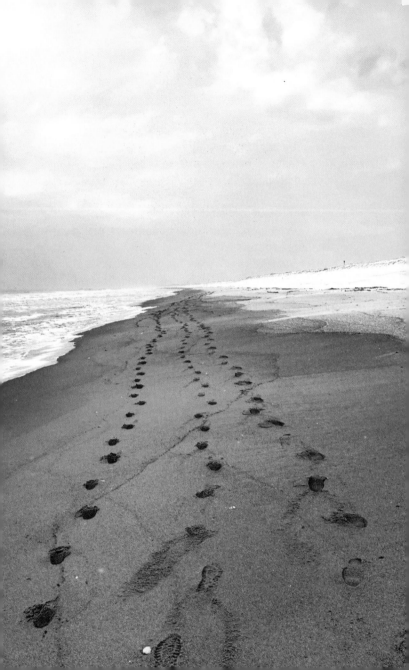

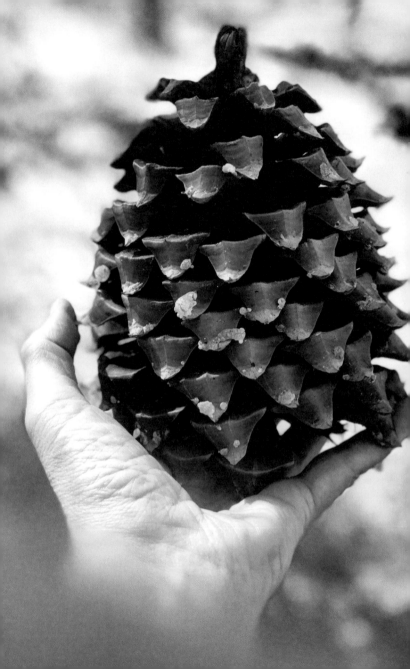

is located in the same part of our brain that affects emotions and memory. In other words, the part of the brain that processes smell interacts with regions in the brain that are responsible for storing emotional memories. That's why scents help us see, remember and place ourselves in a moment.

My walk this morning will forever be associated with the luxurious scents of fog and salt (yes, salt has a fragrance) and the cheerful conversation I had with a friend who joined me. I suspect the next time I go to the beach in the fog I will think of this walk I had today.

Of all the senses, scent is considered the most emotive and primal, and it can transport me into new landscapes that open pathways to unique thinking and creative problem solving. Try this. Close your eyes. Imagine walking in a forest filled with pine trees. Or walking on the sidewalk after the rain. Where does it take you? Who were you with? What else was happening? What do you feel?

Touch

While sight is likely to be the most dominant sense when walking, I have come to profoundly appreciate touch. It is perhaps the sense that almost instantly brings me to the present moment. If I am wearing something that is bothersome or rubbing the wrong way it has the power to transform a walk from glorious to painful. Last week it was incredibly cold and I decided to wear two pairs of socks to be sure that my toes didn't freeze along the way. About a quarter of a mile into the walk all hell broke loose in my left shoe. The socks bunched up, rubbing my toes the wrong way, and I felt the beginnings of a blister. It was wildly annoying. It was too cold to pull my shoes and socks off to make any adjustments so I could either try and ignore it, change my gait to minimise the impact or turn around, go home and start over. At that moment, all three options sounded terrible. I was determined to finish my walk and I was also oddly determined to not let 'something so small' bother me. That wasn't a good idea. By the time I got home I had a sizeable blister, a cranky toe and a bad attitude about my decision. I will say, however, I was very, very present.

When I walk I am almost always wearing a puffy coat, regardless of temperature. I do this for many reasons; the most important is perhaps psychological, not functional. My puffy coat feels like a source of security. Like that moment when someone holds you. Remember as a kid when a loving family member took your hand when you were scared or when you needed it the most, when that person you trusted was there to wrap you up in their arms to create a cocoon that became a safe sanctuary? It's hard to believe a simple coat can evoke such powerful memories, but the touch, the fit, the feeling of the jacket holding me is something that makes me feel braver, safer, stronger — and as if I am not alone on some of my walks. This actually didn't occur to me until one day when I wasn't wearing my coat and I felt almost unbearably exposed. I guess it is a security blanket. Hey, we all need them.

Taste

An added benefit of wearing my puffy coat with pockets brings me to taste. I have started a new practice of often putting a bit of chocolate in my pocket. Chocolate-covered raisins, to be precise. While it might not be an absolute best practice when it comes to nutrition, I find that having a few in my pocket adds a certain rebellious joy, and feels like a wonderful little secret. There is nothing quite like heading into a gnarly headwind and putting my hand in my pocket to find them.

A more subtle experience of taste on a walk happened a few summers ago as I came across a ripe orange grove. As I walked along, I realised that the taste of oranges flavoured my walk. The atmosphere was bright and clean, while the air smelled and tasted like sunshine, vitamin D, citrus and deliciousness.

All of your senses are available to you on a MorningWalk. Invite them to join you. Be curious about each one.

We should take wandering outdoor walks, so that the mind might be nourished and refreshed by the open air and deep breathing.

Seneca

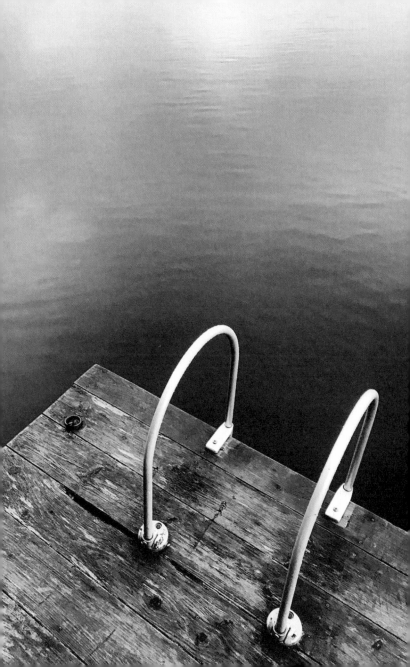

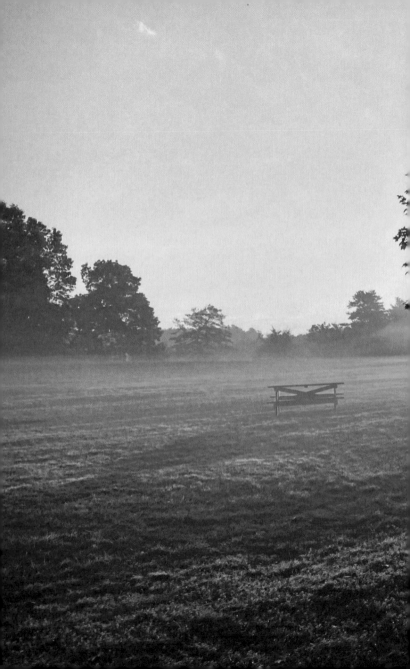

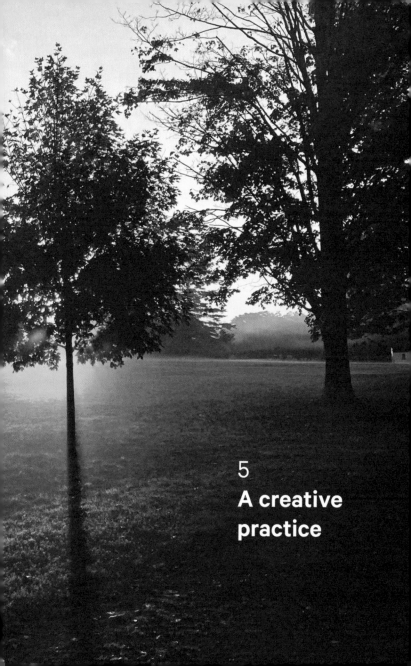

5
**A creative
practice**

Our advertising agency has a big presentation to an important client in a week and we are still working to get to the right idea. As creative director, one of the most terrifying elements of my job is I'm never quite sure when or where The Idea or The Solution may show up. As the days pass, the tension, anxiety and excitement build. There is a complexity to this moment when we start assessing ideas with the team and my feedback goes something like this:

> 'Interesting idea, but not quite there yet.'
> 'Nope.'
> 'Love it, keep going.'
> 'Bananas.'
> 'Great start, however …'
> 'Wonderful, but no.'
> 'Maybe.'
> 'It's a beginning.'
> 'That's crazy, good concept.'

We were getting nowhere fast so I put on my walking shoes and invited my colleagues to join me. I wanted to inspire a collision of conversation and observations, and to unearth and unlock new ways of thinking. I also wanted us to be on an equal footing. No one sat at the head of the table in this meeting. Hierarchy didn't matter. We were aligned and equal in our commitment to find a great idea as we walked through the town.

In all honesty, half the walk was play, colleagues telling stories, enjoying the sun, teasing one another; the other half was focused, directed problem-solving. The play part of the walk was essential to our ability to generate new ideas and unexpected solutions. Play is required for creativity and walking helps place people in an atmosphere more conducive to productive fun and games than sitting at a desk. I remember hearing that eureka moments often happen in the subconscious when we aren't narrowly thinking about the problem at hand. That is why we often hear about people coming up with the idea whilst in the shower or cooking breakfast.

During the walk we generated many new thoughts and directions. Half of them were terrible and unusable but made us laugh. The other half were a result of working through the process of getting the bad ideas out of the way. Perhaps more importantly we were a team: our shared focus and our environment inspired a new way of thinking, together.

The truth of the matter is there is no surefire or guaranteed process for unearthing a great idea. At the end of the day, it is trust in the team and, I believe, the addition of movement that shape unique and innovative thinking.

Creativity requires us to see things anew, and for me, the most powerful innovation tool is walking. A Stanford University research report by Oppezzo and Schwartz concluded, 'Walking led to an increase in analogical creativity ... walking has a very specific benefit — the improvement of creativity.'

Walking awakens the senses and forces the brain to use multiple parts. Significant and disparate areas of the brain are needed to coordinate movements and to maintain balance while walking. This movement stimulates areas of the brain that are generally not all lit up at the same time. In the Stanford study cited above, it was found that walking boosts creative output by 60 percent. We are unconsciously competent when it comes to walking. We don't need to think about putting one foot in front of the other. We get to take advantage of the fact that the brain is fully engaged in a way that ignites creativity.

An interesting academic article by Leisman, Moustafa and Shafir, three brain scientists, published in *Frontiers in Public Health*, summarised by Nicole Dean in *Brain World Magazine*, suggests that 'complex human cognition, including our remarkable capacity for innovation, developed right along with the ability to walk ... Granted, when we go for a walk, the very brain structures that allow us to walk also allow us to access our most sophisticated cognitive abilities.'

One could argue that our ability as a species to problem-solve, innovate and create stems from our ability to walk. Many well-known pioneers have used walking as a key tool. Steve Jobs is noted for having conducted 'Walk and Talks' with friends, colleagues and employees. He thought they were essential to the creation of some of Apple's most important insights and successful products. The power and connection from a walk don't just happen with people who are familiar with one another. As Minda Zetlin wrote in a 2020 *Inc.* article: 'Conducting a meeting while walking has clear health benefits for the participants, and as it turns out, it benefits the meeting, too. New research from the University of Hong Kong shows that walking side by side helps people connect to each other.' The power of synchronised steps, arm movement and breathing is thought to build a bond without even having to say a word.

As a result, many influential thought leaders have said that walking is an essential daily ritual. It seems to me I am in good company. Here are a few:

William Wordsworth
Henry David Thoreau
Albert Einstein
Oprah Winfrey
Charles Darwin
Virginia Woolf
Isaac Asimov
John Muir
Ludwig van Beethoven
Mahatma Gandhi
Sigmund Freud
and
Edward Payson Weston
the godfather of the pedestrianism movement.

I believe the reason walking is such a powerful tool for creativity is the juxtaposition of something that is elusive and ephemeral — an idea — with something so foundational and physical — walking. The more I move, the more I am moved.

Nature's particular gift to the walker ...
is to set the mind jogging, to make it
garrulous, exalted, a little mad maybe —
certainly creative and suprasensitive,
until at last, it really seems to be outside
of you and as if it were talking to you
whilst you are talking back to it.
... here and now, the mind has shaken
off its harness, is snorting and kicking
up heels like a colt in a meadow.

Kenneth Grahame

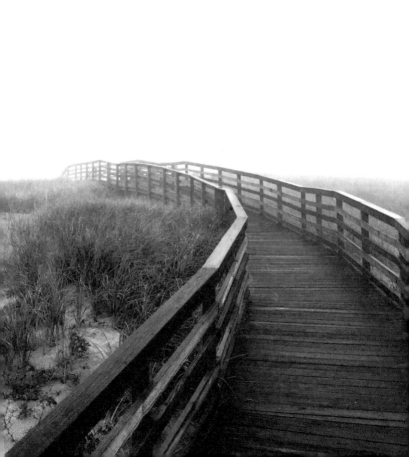

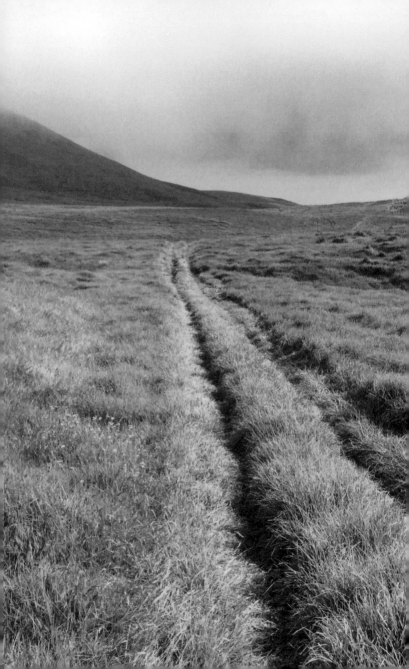

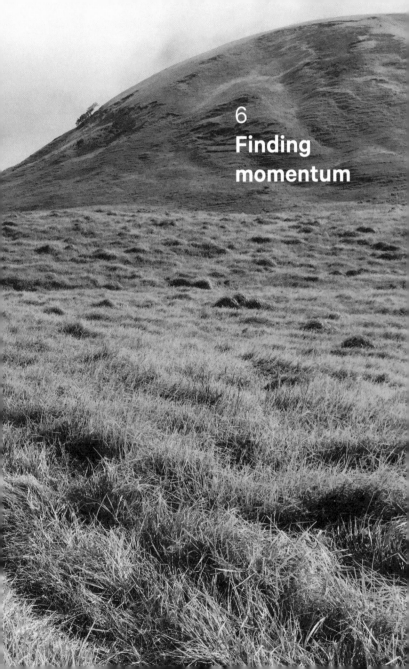

6
**Finding
momentum**

Up before any sunlight, no alarm.
Shoes, headlamp and warm cozies on.
Set an intention for the walk. Patience.
Head out the door.
Tea when I get home.

It's blowing like stink. The rain seems to find every little
opening to seep in and my hat brim drips, drips, drips.
By the time I have finished 9 miles I am soaked to the
bones, despite having fine-tuned my gear and layers.
Thankfully, I was warm. If I begin down the path of getting
cold, uncertainty and fear creep in. Feeling warm makes
these walks feel heroic rather than threatening. I feel safe
when I am warm. As I walk, a rebellious voice visits.

> *'You are getting over a sore throat, no need to stay out.'*
> *'You've gone long enough, sweetheart.'*
> *'Tea would taste so much better than rain.'*

I have been in this situation many times over the past
years and I recognise this voice. She can be convincing
and charming, seductive in her attempts to take me home.
Experience has taught me when it's too cold, too wet, too
hot or humid, that's when endorphins explode, problems
get solved and true healing begins. The experience of
being out in challenging weather fuels a kind of self-
righteous pride that creates momentum. Looking back
over nearly a decade of daily walks, the days where
I almost talk myself out of doing it are the days that
MorningWalk has the most impact.

I am often asked, 'How do you do it every day?' 'Where do you find the momentum?'

I must admit that on that first walk years ago I had no idea that I would still be walking every day. The desire then was more immediate, more urgent. To spend more time outdoors. So how do I still do it every day? It is easy. I have discovered that some of the most meaningful lessons are the subtle learnings that can only be understood over time. I do it every day because MorningWalk has become a classroom. An intimate school that teaches me about myself. It is also part of my identity: I am someone who walks every morning. Just as someone who runs most days thinks of themselves as a runner, or someone who paints each day thinks of themselves as a painter. I walk every day — I am a walker. The idea of not doing it feels like an act of self-betrayal.

Here are a few of the lessons I have learned along the way.

No two walks are alike

Even if many of the variables are the same, each walk is wildly and beautifully different. Every walk brings a new story, a new lesson, a new view and an opportunity to understand the world in a unique way. I look at each walk as a clean slate, a blank page.

There is delight to be found in each walk
Even when the weather stings with icy rain or I have a bad case of the grumps, there is always something in the walk that is absolutely wonderful: the gratitude for a cosy warm hat, the courageous feeling of being out when your inner voice told you to stay in bed, the view of the trees with their soaked bark contrasting with the snow on the branches, a generous conversation with a friend, the satisfaction of having walked 3,285 days in a row.

This too shall pass
Emotions and thoughts, much like the weather, will have their moment and then move on. Every walk has a beginning and an end. The tide will come and go. The seasons will change. The sun will rise, then set. All the junk in your head will roll in, then roll out.

There is no such thing as bad weather ...
... just unsuitable clothing, as the legendary Lake District walker Alfred Wainwright once wrote. Quite a few walks happen in what might be considered unfriendly weather. Make sure your kit is complete so that you will be comfortable.

Discipline is a reward in itself
When you have done something for 30 days in a row, it's hard to find a reason to break that streak. Commitment is hard, but habit is powerful. This is why it is imperative to just keep going. One foot in front of the other.

Stay grounded and look up
A good reminder: feet on the ground, eyes to the sky.

There is essential information in the quiet

Our inner world needs our attention. At the start of the covid-19 pandemic, I found that I didn't want to listen to anything related to the news and allowed myself periods of silence to feel more at peace. I took the earbuds out and discovered that I had been missing a lot by distracting myself with external information. Be sure to give yourself periods of silence.

Disconnect to reconnect

Most walks I take by myself. It is an opportunity to quiet the external noise of culture and expectation and listen to my instinct, my gut, my essential nature. In that way, every walk is an adventure. An adventure of thoughts, of internal weather, of new trails. Each walk is a personal pilgrimage.

Emotions need motion

There are days when unexpected emotions pop up, and it's hard to pinpoint exactly what I am feeling. Adding motion to those moments is a very helpful way to identify what and where the feeling lives, and its source.

There's a reason why the words 'motion' and 'emotion' are so similar. Motion comes from the Latin *movere*, to move; emotion comes from *emovere*, to disturb. So we shouldn't be surprised when motion stimulates the emotions.

Take action, every day

Put simply, commit to yourself. Walking each day has the potential to change your life. It happens slowly, deliberately. Commitment is walk by walk, step by step.

You don't need much

It *is* that simple.

Whatever walking looks like for you — leisurely and slow or vibrant and determined; in nature or in your urban neighbourhood — I encourage you to get creative and find a new way of embedding it into your daily schedule. Walking is a mindset, not simply an action. Include it in what you already do. This is a surefire way to build and maintain a life where walking is a vital part of your day. If you build momentum towards a goal, then at some point you won't want to break the streak. Here are a few thoughts on how to embed walking into your day.

1. Plan a walking meeting

2. Park as far away from your front door/place of work as possible

3. Make your coffee date a walking coffee date

4. Walk part of the way to work or to a friend's house

5. Get off the train/subway/bus one stop early

6. Organise a walking book group

7. Take micro-adventures and walk down a new street every day

8. Try 'plogging' (picking up trash while jogging/walking)

9. Take the stairs, not the lift

10. Start a walking challenge with family, neighbours, colleagues or friends, even if you don't live in the same area. Create a hashtag and get walking.

11. Keep walking shoes handy (in your car/under your desk/by the back door)

12. Consider a wearable fitness app to track your steps and have fun with the data

13. Adopt a dog! Or offer to take a friend's dog for a walk

Part of the momentum and ongoing motivation to continue comes from having done it so regularly. Energy creates energy. Yes, walking every day is essential to me, but I don't do it just for myself. I do it for those who are around me. I believe we show up in the world with more clarity, intelligent energy, and self-awareness when we create the space to tend to our own wellbeing: mental, physical, emotional and spiritual. The personal commitment is nourishing but, perhaps most importantly, those who surround me feel the influence. That motivates me.

So, while my MorningWalk is essentially an individual and intimate mindfulness practice, I also see the impact this has on my little world. I am more likely to have the perspective and energy I want for the day ahead after having gone for a walk. A good friend used to have a small sign in her office which said something along the lines of, 'Please take responsibility for the energy you bring into this space.' Every time I read it, I knew that I was more likely to show up with the energy I could be proud of after having gone for a walk. When I am upset about something or my buttons have been pushed, I am better able to take responsibility for how I show up *after* MorningWalk because I have spent that time observing my own beliefs, thoughts and expectations.

Am I changing the world with a walk each day? No, but I do think we are responsible for the perspectives and enthusiasm we cultivate in ourselves and for the energy we bring to the world. Is a MorningWalk a miracle cure? Certainly not. Is the energy I show up with always as I intend? Hell, no. Does a MorningWalk start my day off on the right foot and get it moving in the right direction? Yes.

When I first started MorningWalk I used to say to my friends and family, 'Please don't take anything I say seriously until I have been for a walk.' This is still true.

If you are in a bad mood, go for a walk. If you are still in a bad mood, go for another walk.

—

Hippocrates

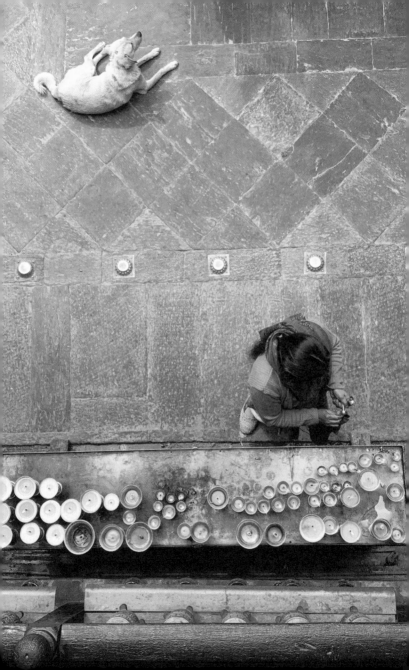

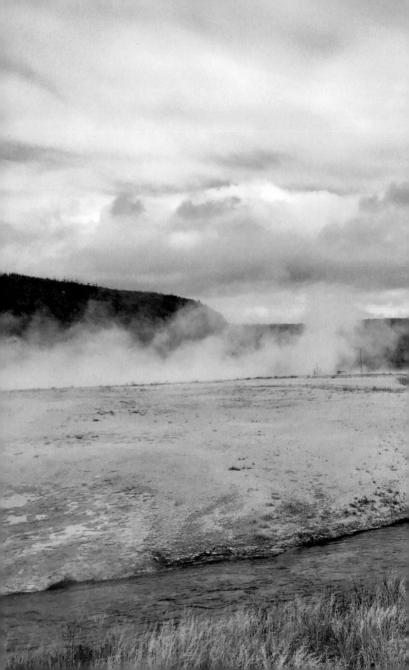

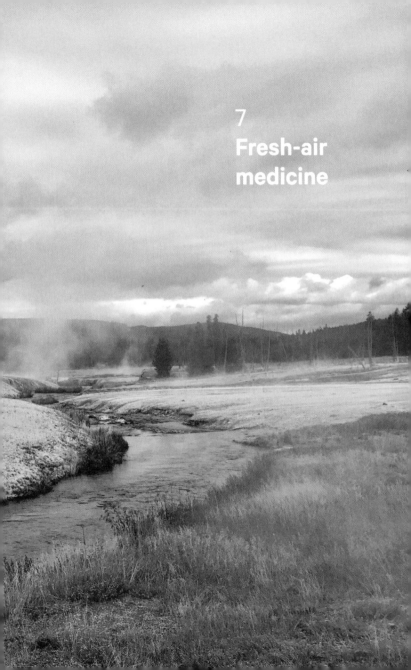

7
Fresh-air medicine

For the first time in nine years, I almost successfully talked myself out of going for a walk. On this morning, the state of the world felt too heavy, too much to carry. I didn't have an emotional backpack big enough to hold all of my feelings. They were too much, too raw, too prickly, too weighty. The conversation in my head went like this:

VOICE: *'Sister, stay in bed. Rest.'*

ME: *'What? Say that again.*
Really, I can stay in bed today?'

VOICE: *'Of course, you have never missed a day.*
Give yourself a break.
Let your body be quiet, unmoving.'

ME: *'But I feel like crap and I know that*
putting on my walking shoes always
makes everything better.
There has never been a day where
I went for a walk and things didn't feel
physically better or my thoughts clearer.'

VOICE: *'Sure, but it isn't required.'*

ME: *'Thank you. I'm going for a walk.'*

There have been times when a MorningWalk has been a confidante, a coach, a therapist and a best friend all in one. It all starts with the first step. For example, when faced with a business challenge that nearly took me down, I needed a way to sort it out. The issue required dedicated time to look at the situation from all sides, to make sure that I understood all the possible perspectives and the potential solutions. I decided that for the next week I would dedicate each walk to this situation and see what showed up. There was no predetermined destination or outcome for each walk, only the desire to understand the situation more fully. By the end of the week I was clear-minded and knew exactly what to do next. You have to walk the miles to experience that.

Thankfully, moving our body produces life's most natural and effective anti-depressants. The mind, body and spirit are a whole. Mental health is brain health and brain health is physical health. Taking consistent action is the only possible way to move towards this holistic wellbeing — and a MorningWalk is fuel. Someone once said to me, 'The reason regular exercise matters is because it trains your brain to believe that your effort matters.' It changes our brain and therefore how we look at our life.

During the pandemic of 2020 and 2021, walking became a crucial form of preventive healing. Perhaps it was always about healing, but I'm not sure I would have used that word a few years ago. MorningWalk felt like medicine. A way to walk towards the beauty of the day and away from things that no longer served me. It is both a mindset and a practice that has brought me endless comfort. Interestingly, doctors are now prescribing a walk in a natural setting to improve mood, and ease levels of anxiety, stress and depression. Nature bathing or forest bathing (Shinrin-yoku) has been shown to have quite a profound impact on mood. In a study published by the Japanese *Environmental Health and Preventive Medicine* journal, it was suggested that forest bathing and walks outside 'can lead to improvements in physiological and psychological health in people of working age, as demonstrated by the decrease in blood pressure and the alleviation of negative psychological parameters'. Go find some trees and walk amongst them, whether a forest, park, tree-lined street, or a single tree near you. There is solace in knowing this 'prescription' for healing.

Walking in the dark

Walks in the dark are perhaps my most magical and medicinal walks. There is something about dimming one of our senses that makes the other senses brighter. In the winter months, most of my walks start in the dark. The earth is quieter, the pace of everything is tender. Lights coming on in kitchens. People wrapped in robes collecting newspapers. Dogs walking their owners. There is nothing like the intimate connected feeling of my community waking up. I am lucky; I am able to walk in a place I am very familiar with and where I feel secure.

As the sun gets ready to peek above the horizon, there is already a community up and awake. I see the same people every day. The runner with the beautiful gait, the walker with the blinking wristband, the brothers out on their morning bike ride. It feels as if we are part of a discreet club that knows the opportunity and grace of the morning. I don't know anyone's name or where they live but somehow, we are connected. Connected by the commitment to the morning, and I like to think, a commitment to each other as we go about our separate rituals, together.

Just recently, I went out on a snowy, winter walk with a small group of friends. It wasn't a sunrise walk; instead we headed out after the sun had set at 4:30pm. It was already dark so we switched on our headlamps as we walked through a hallway of winter rhododendrons. At one point, almost instinctively, we all became very quiet. We stopped our conversation, stopped walking and turned off our headlamps. The moment felt as if we had just walked into a sacred, candlelit cathedral. We paused and collectively took a deep, cold breath. In the darkest of dark frigid New England winters, we were in the shadow of the moon, inspired and together. It was an instant, yet it felt monumental. Walking in the dark makes the world feel more dramatic, intimate, even cinematic.

Adaptability

You'd be surprised who you meet in the early morning as the sun begins to rise. Birdwatchers. As it turns out, the location where I walk is on a migratory path for many birds: bald eagles, snowy owls, peregrine falcons, and the elegant American goldfinch. As a group, birdwatchers are some of the most enthusiastic and generous souls on the planet.

One of the key lessons from birdwatchers and the birds themselves is the ability to adapt and to modify behaviour. The ability to adapt to changing environments and circumstances is a mighty lesson. This was perhaps one of the most difficult lessons for me to embrace and embody fully. Adaptability is not a casual lesson. It is one that requires gentle yet constant attention. Thankfully, MorningWalk is a classroom that I enter every single morning, and the teacher is unrelenting and beautiful: Mama Nature, the true teacher.

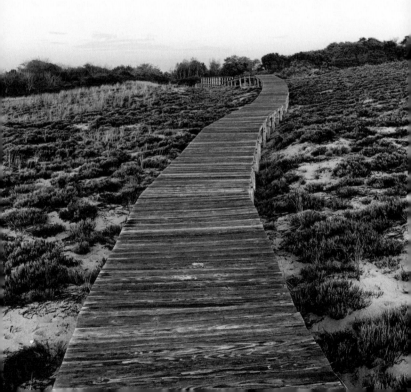

Above all, do not lose your desire to walk:
Every day I walk myself into a state of
wellbeing and walk away from every illness;
I have walked myself into my best thoughts,
and I know of no thought so burdensome
that one cannot walk away from it.

Søren Kierkegaard

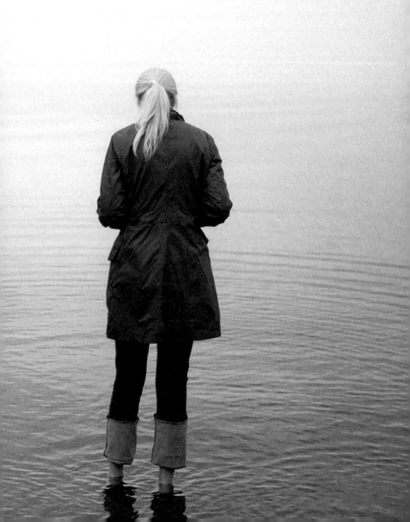

8
A way
of being

I received some news that was very difficult. Life-alteringly, intimately difficult. The ultimate betrayal. As I left the office that afternoon, I told myself that I could either go home and curl up in bed to try and feel better, or, I could walk. I went home, put on my shoes and set out to do my familiar loop of 7.3 miles. I walked through the night. All. Night. Step by painful step. I needed to keep walking.

Each lap held a different emotion. There was big anger, wild frustration, bold denial, pure rage, broken trust—sometimes all at once. Each lap became an elegant chapter about grieving, about reflection, about pain, about finding my way back to myself. I stayed out until sunrise, went home, took a shower and walked to work.

Each one of those steps was essential to seeing clearly. Understanding what had happened. I somehow needed to find comfort in the discomfort. I needed to find my way, myself. The pain wasn't meant to be avoided. It was meant to be understood, and my way to understand it was to walk. As Ram Dass, teacher and poet, said, 'We're all just walking each other home.' I was walking myself home. And truth be told, walking all night saved me.

A friend once said, 'The "daily" part of a daily commitment is hard, near impossible sometimes.' I never would have imagined myself choosing to walk through the night as a way to heal what felt like a mortal wound but years of putting one foot in front of the other had taught me to trust the discipline of the practice. I knew in my gut that walking was exactly what I needed. I could only find my way home by walking.

At this point you may find yourself asking, 'How do I make this a way of life? How do I keep going and trust in the practice?'

A way forward

As we saw earlier (pages 34–35), there are things you can do to start a daily walking practice. However, as time goes on, you will begin to find places where it feels difficult. Think about how to solve those issues. For me, when I wake up, for some odd reason my feet always feel cold. It was a psychological deterrent in the colder months because my mind told me I was just going to get colder and more uncomfortable. So I found some super-cosy slippers to get me from my bed to my walking shoes and in the winter I now wear heated socks. The space between waking and walking is a tender place. I needed tools, tricks, hacks and solutions to make sure there wasn't a reason to not go.

Connect your new habit to an existing one so that anchor will help trigger your new habit. The idea is to make the new behaviour automatic. I put my walking shoes out each night so I can't miss them, right in front of the sink where my toothbrush is perched.

When your thoughts say, 'There is no way I can do that,' consider responding with, 'But just imagine if I could'. Also, remember, there won't be an immediate impact— let the habit be the goal.

On your walk, remember to relax and tap into all of your senses. The sound of the city waking up, the smell of the pine trees, the feel of fine dust in your shoes, the lights coming on in your neighbours' houses, the sound of the local train leaving the station; all points of inspiration to get you out the door.

Lastly, give yourself a compliment. Every day. One of my sons taught me this. We were out skiing one day, headed down a very steep hill, when I overheard him singing to himself. When we got to the bottom I asked him what was up. He replied, 'Well, it was a little intimidating going down

so I decided to sing compliments to myself the whole way.'
This is a practice we can all embrace. Try it!

Part of MorningWalk becoming a way of life for me was
being generous in how I looked at the practice. There have
been days, when I was travelling or sick, when the distance
I covered was a walk around the block rather than several
miles. For me that required a kindness in my definition.
It isn't about distance, or speed, or time; therefore, any
intentional walk fits into my expectation of a MorningWalk.
It is about thoughtfully engaging with your morning.

**So, what are you going to do with this
new year? With these 365 days? Every one
of them full of 24 hours of opportunity.
Each day full of 86,400 seconds.
About the same number of heartbeats.**

Mark Shayler

MorningWalk is my fuel source. It does not deplete or
drain the momentum I have for the day; rather it creates,
builds and magnifies energy. I know that walking in the
morning helps me to be present and productive. While
productivity isn't a specific goal, having the energy to be
attentive, organised, thoughtful, caring and creative is.
That's productive. I often hear people say, 'But I'm too tired
to go for a walk/run/workout.' While I understand that
feeling, the truth of the matter is walking creates more
energy. Try it. Go for a walk when you are really tired.
See what happens. It's amazing what a simple walk can do.

That moment of waking is an incredible opportunity, and it's quite a tragedy if you go straight to your to-do list.

David Whyte

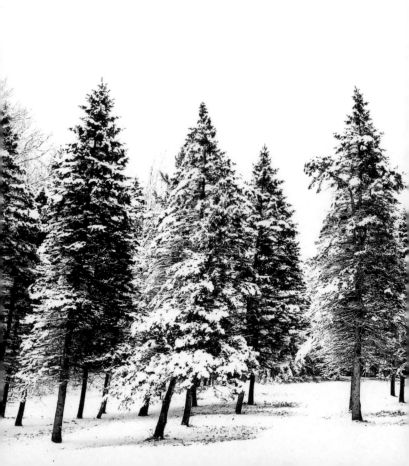

9
Keep going

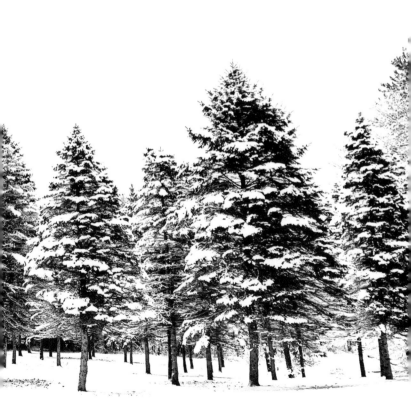

Good morning, New Year. Just returned from a very, very long and beautiful walk. Twelve miles, about three hours. It was gorgeous. Bright. Calm. Cold. It all felt so hopeful and nourishing. I didn't want to come in. I wanted to breathe in the sunlight and the birdsong. I used the space around me to discard the negative voices in my head from last year. Left along the side of the road are all those distracting unhelpful thoughts that worked their way into my mind: 'You aren't — enough.' 'You are too —.' 'Why did you say —?' Blah, blah, blah. As I walk it is easier and easier to leave these stories behind and what remains? A brilliant, sparkly day, abundant with accompanying gratitude.

Walk. Breathe in. Breathe out.
Notice everything. Notice this day.

Halfway through today's walk I came upon a snowy owl — a rare sight and a pure pleasure. In the past, I would have missed it. Life can be so busy we overlook what is right in front of us. Today is different. Years of practice have taught me to slow down and look up. As I walked past the snowy owl, she took off, circled around and landed just up the road, almost as if to say, 'Come on, keep going.'

Walking in the morning is the equivalent of writing a daily journal. It's a place to be with thoughts of the day. There are going to be days where you don't feel like writing/walking. Do it anyway. There may be a day where you forget to do it in the morning. Do it in the evening instead. You may decide walking is too time-consuming. Walk anyway. The lessons arrive when you commit to it and do the work. Go for the walk. Remember, it doesn't matter how far or how fast you walk. What matters is that you went. MorningWalk is the practice of commitment, of breath, of attention, of trust, of humility, of generosity, of patience, of discipline, of discovery, of pure happiness, of hope and of love. A walk is building resilience, loving your body, committing to your wellbeing and taking action. It's a radical act of self-care.

The other day I woke up with a tightness in my chest. It was worry, fear and a splash of negative thinking. As I got up, the wonderful thought I had was, 'Thank goodness for the walk I am about to take.' There is something about a walk that feels like a gentle massage for your entire body and spirit. I remember when I first started this practice I would visualise every muscle, every cell, every element of my body getting a massage. It's like holding a baby and instinctively starting to rock back and forth from one foot to the other. It's a dance of care, soothing — and it is wonderfully calming, I suspect, to both the person holding and the baby. Gentle movement with a familiar pace. Walking has a similar feel and tempo. The rhythm of two steps per breath feels like comfort, certainty and love. I have found that, during the pandemic especially, walking with a focus on my breathing helped me to feel more in control of my life.

Another beautiful thing about walking is that it doesn't require a membership, a monthly pass or a sign-up sheet. Simply put on your shoes and walk out the door: find a street, field, sidewalk, hiking trail, bike path, backyard, front yard, local park, back road, long route to your friend's house ... and go. If you're in a wheelchair, there are likely some routes that are more welcoming. MorningWalk can shift to adapt to what you have going on each day. This was one of the critical elements that made this practice doable for me. I could cut the walk short or start an hour early should other things in my day require attention and time. There were some days when I needed an extra hour to prepare something for work and I would simply shorten the walk. Or if I was feeling sick I would wait until the sun came up and slowly walk around the neighbourhood.

Walking may not be a powerful aerobic workout but it is perhaps the most powerful and injury-free form of exercise around. There is no shortage of scientific research to back up the effectiveness of adding walking to your routine. One study found that 10 to 12 minutes of walking increased self-confidence, mood and attentiveness. And, as we've already seen, walking in nature significantly reduces negative thoughts and improves brain health. Walking is a superpower. No question.

It is only when we are well rested, clear-headed and open to what is coming next that our life becomes a true reflection of what we want it to be. Walking is the perfect way to get there, by exploring the world and allowing space for dreaming bigger. And it has helped me add energy to those dreams.

Walking is the ultimate navigational tool. It helps us to navigate the earth, and our life, ultimately helping us see who we are and where we want to go. When a walk gets hard or cold or feels too long, how do you weather the storm? The lesson always remains the same. Keep going. This answer is just around the corner. What is uncomfortable or unclear now will not last forever. Literally step by step you get closer to the top of the hill, to home, to being warmed up, to being done. Walking is a mirror for what happens in life. Some days are harder than others, some hills are steeper than others, but fundamentally the way to get through or to the top is to break it down into small actions. Walking is a joyful and sometimes comedic endeavour with plenty to teach if you can stay attentive to things like turkeys. Yes, turkeys.

Lessons from turkeys

On my favourite loop, more often than not I see a flock of 20 turkeys. All the turkeys I run into are arrogant. They hang out in the middle of the road. They perch in the big oak trees 30 feet in the air as if they can really fly. They can't, really. But they think they can (don't come at me, ornithologists...). They are constantly talking and the male turkeys think they are something special, always flaunting their plumage and parading around as if they own the place. It's fair to say we have spent a lot of time looking at each other. Turkeys are unlikely philosophers, but honestly, I feel I have learned a lot from them. I am not an ornithologist. I am not even an honest birdwatcher, however, just by being with the flock and watching how they interact over the course of many years, I think I may have learned a few things: be wildly confident, empower others to lead, over communicate, own it, strut your stuff unapologetically, get up, get to it and keep going.

Get up and get to it

Motivation is a choice and it has sparkly magic in it. When motivated to show up for yourself, you are also showing up for other people in your life. Motivation isn't an intangible energy that just appears out of nowhere. It is a force that compels us to take action and it is necessary to help us navigate life. It feels like active invisible inspiration.

I have often wondered where motivation comes from. Does it come before an activity or after? Is it the cause or the result? Perhaps it is both. When I first started walking, there were days when I would need a splash of motivation to head out the door — some days more than others. It is also true that when I returned, I would feel as if I had all the motivation that I would need for the coming year. Now, years later, I find that once I am awake and out of bed, I can't help but go for a walk because I know the impact it will have on my day. As Steven Pressfield said in his book *The War of Art*, 'At some point, the pain of not doing it becomes greater than the pain of doing it.' He was referring to writing, not walking, but the point still stands.

A MorningWalk each day is also a way for me to plot a secure way forward. Knowing that the sun will rise, I will put on my shoes and go for a walk. I can trust that and, as a result, I can trust the future. It's a powerful and comforting thought — and feels like an invitation to believe in our

ability to design tomorrow. Because the world has yet
to wake up when I set out, the day feels like it is for me
to define.

> **I've always liked the time before dawn
> because there's no one around to remind
> me who I'm supposed to be so it's easier
> to remember who I am.**

> Brian Andreas

Mornings are a gorgeous blank page. There is a profound
sense of freedom to create the day as we want. It is
undoubtedly too strong a statement to say MorningWalk
has become an artful act, but it certainly is a ritual of
creativity, expression, beauty, and some days one of pure
exuberance. It has become a way to start the day feeling
the aliveness in the world with an open sense of possibility.
In each walk, anything is possible and everything is
beautiful, even in the cold, grumpy, icy rain. MorningWalk
is a desire to observe beauty. To be with beauty. To make
things beautiful. I guess it is an artful act.

The beginner's mind

Walking the earth is an essential way to measure and see
ourselves in the world. To view the world in multiple ways
is to begin to understand it. Each walk provides us with
unique and important information, essential to navigating
our days with a richness and wonder. New experiences
are the teachers. Learning expands our appreciation of
the world. Walking every day is a way to guarantee that
we have the opportunity and raw material for learning

in each day. Events that require us to be a beginner are essential for growth. The beginner's mind is a humbling and mighty tool.

Amateurs with a beginner's mind pursue their study, practice or endeavour because they love doing it. It's that simple. It is the pursuit of beauty, truth, excitement and love. In fact, the Latin word *amator* means lover. We amateurs are willing to navigate the tumult, chaos and humility of being a beginner: the learning, the failing, the practising, the struggling, the questioning, in order to understand the lesson.

According to the Zen teacher Shunryu Suzuki, 'In the Beginner's Mind there are many possibilities. In the Expert's Mind, there are few.' I would argue that the spirit of the amateur and the practice of developing a beginner's mind are exactly what walking is all about: take one step at a time, live without 'shoulds', let go of your knowing, experience the moment fully, forget common sense, ignore fear of failure or the excitement of success, listen for questions, not answers, be open to anything that may come into view. Move and learn with awe, regardless of success, weather, mood, accomplishment or achievement. This is the gift of the beginner. Every day on MorningWalk you have an opportunity to start over.

In my early twenties, I was told that the best way to predict your future was to create it. I was never really sure what that meant. Honestly, I'm not sure I know now. What I do know is that MorningWalk enables me to get honest with myself in terms of how I would like that future to look. There is an opportunity in creating a habit that is so regular you don't even think about it. That regularity allows the mind to explore the moment and humbly learn. I don't have anywhere to go, anywhere to be, or any expectation of an outcome. The lesson is having done the walk, not in walking. The body carries information and the answers to our day are inside us; walking wakes them up. Sometimes the world is so loud, we can't hear. Or we are so sure of the stories in our head, we don't believe what is embedded in us. The humility of the beginner's mind is a key to unlock the possibilities of that inner life.

Teachers of meditation will say that a practice can be done sitting, standing, walking or lying down. MorningWalk is meditation, a commitment to an inner life. It is a practice where we hold space, listen, observe and eventually, find our story. MorningWalk goes beyond the transactional and physical elements of walking. It doesn't matter where you go, only that you learn something in the journey. There is no destination — there is no 'there' to get to. The idea that I am not going anywhere yet have travelled so far is essential to MorningWalk. We may think the practice is taking us somewhere, but really it is the present moment, one right after the other. We each get to decide which path, for how long, and where the walk will take us.

Ultimately, MorningWalk is about love. Love for the planet. Love for the bend in the road. Love for the ability to do it. Love for bumping into friends along the way. Love for the blistering humidity. Love for the cold toes. Love for the time together. Love for the solitude. Love for the warm drink after. Love for the ability to move. Love for the space to think and just be. MorningWalk is about love. Period.

I will arise and go now.

William Butler Yeats

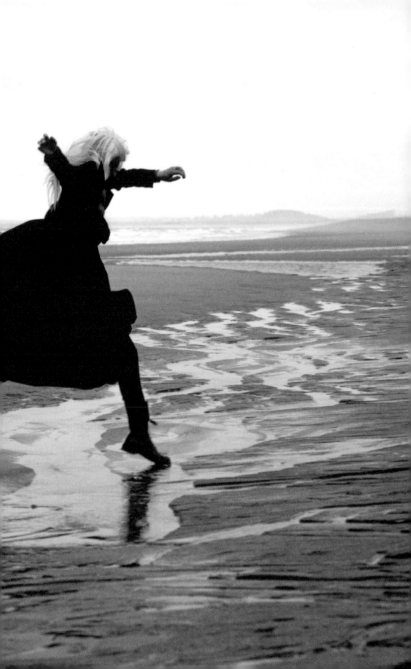

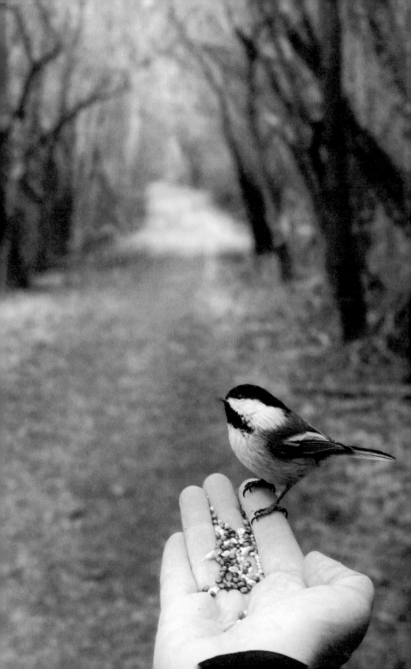

Walking mantra

May you find happiness in walking;
May you find joy in walking;
May you find energy in walking;
May you find answers in walking;
May you find beauty in walking;
May you find a sparkly world in walking;
May you find right now in walking;
May you find peace in walking;
May you find bravery in walking;
May you find love in walking.

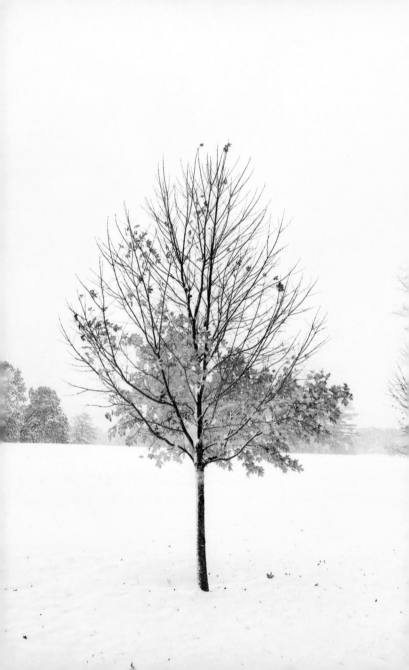

FAQ

Here are some of the questions that I am asked quite regularly, so I thought they would be useful to share.

How many miles is your MorningWalk?
On average 8 to 10 miles, but honestly the mileage doesn't matter.

What time do you usually walk?
I am generally out the door around 5am.

With such an early start, what time do you need to get to sleep?
Between 8–9pm (I realise this won't work for everybody!)

Do you ever get scared walking in the dark alone?
I don't. I would recommend, however, that when going out for a walk you let someone else know where you will be and consider taking a whistle or some other alarm with you.

Do you prefer walking alone or walking with others?
I need to walk by myself a majority of the time, but I love, love, love having company. During the pandemic, it was my primary way to socialise with friends.

What are your key pieces of gear?
My headlamp and good running/walking shoes.
(Also see Chapter 2)

How do you decide on a route?
There isn't a science or logic to it. Honestly, it is a bit of serendipity with a splash of convenience.

Why did you start when you did? Did you set out with a specific goal in mind a decade ago or did you just start walking?
My goal was simple: to spend more time outdoors. I realised that was where I was happiest and so I needed to build that into my day. It has evolved into something essential.

Do you ever walk barefoot?
Sometimes *(see Chapter 3)*. I have come to realise that taking care of my feet is critical and walking barefoot is part of that regime.

How do you keep at it?
It has become easier over time. Every walk is a good walk. Things are always better after walking.

What are your favourite things to listen to?
I listen to music, podcasts and books about half of the time and the other half is internal work.

How fast do you normally walk?
I don't keep track, but I do 8 miles in about 2 hours. Roughly.

What's your preferred brand of footwear?
I wear Hoka One One Bondis (not an ad — I genuinely get asked this!) and I have a pair specifically for the winter that are half a size too big to allow for an extra pair of socks.

Do you carry a camera?
No, I use my phone camera.

Do you do any other workouts?
Firstly, I don't consider MorningWalk a workout, although every now and again I will combine a little running and walking on my MorningWalk — it just feels great to get the heart rate up. As far as other workouts go, sometimes I hop on an ergometer (rowing machine). I spent many years as a competitive rower, so getting on the erg is a wonderful reminder of when I was very fit.

Does time of day matter?
For me, first thing in the morning is the most impactful time of day. I love being present as the world wakes up. To start my day with a few hours outdoors where I feel most at home has become an essential way to take care of myself. But if it works for you, MorningWalk can happen in the afternoon or evening. It is a mindset.

Do you have a favourite season to walk in?
Autumn/fall because I love the warm breezes, there's no humidity and everything is ripe: tomatoes and cornflowers. This season feels like a hug.

How cold does it have to get for you not to go?
I always go. Over time, I have found the right gear to inspire me to always go. Part of this practice was to overcome resistance.

If you ever had to miss a day, how do you think you would feel? Is the 'undefeated' feeling part of it?
I haven't missed a day, so I really don't know. There have certainly been very short walks, around the block, for example, when I've felt unwell. Is feeling 'undefeated' part of it? I don't think so, instead my impetus is 'always go'. The familiar routine is a very grounding feeling.

What are the top three things you've learned about forming and maintaining habits?
1. Making a commitment to yourself and following through is the ultimate in love
2. Meaningful habits happen step by step, not all at once
3. Habits are powerful because they create neurological cravings

Do you ever walk without your phone?
I always have my phone because I take a photo each day as a visual diary and an act of accountability. Also, it makes sense from a safety point of view.

Where did your Instagram handle @parkhere come from?
My middle name is Park.

Do you eat before you walk or bring some food with you?
I don't, but that is simply because I go out so early in the morning. When I get home the first thing I do is make a cup of tea.

What changes when you're away from home?
The first thing I do when I am in a new location is look for a walking route. Often I will use an app called AllTrails. (I also love iNaturalist when I am out and about for the

identification of plants, birds and bugs. This app allows you to tap into a community of naturalists.)

What has been your longest walk?
My longest walk was over the course of three days: 25 miles a day. It was to raise money for breast cancer research. We started in Framingham, MA and ended in Boston.

Do you do the same route every day?
I have about half a dozen routes I do regularly. I actually like the repetition because it feels familiar and friendly.

What is the most surprising benefit you've found on your walks?
How waking up and immediately adding energy to the day impacts the whole day.

Do you set a specific intention for each walk?
Honestly, I intend to, however in reality some days it is all about walking the grumpies out or attending to a creative question.

What is your favourite MorningWalk?
Sunrise walk, by myself, on New Year's Day each year. I feel such optimism and clarity in that moment.

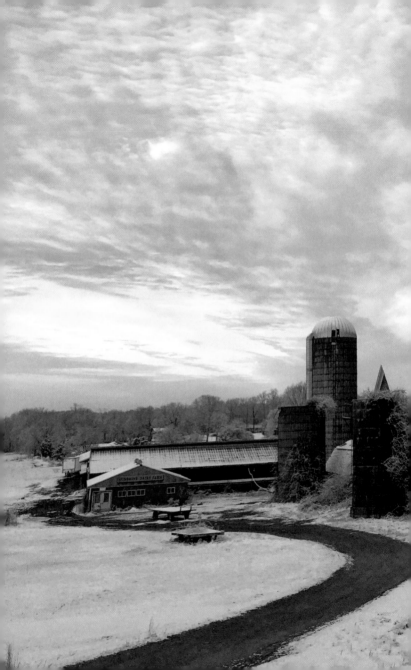

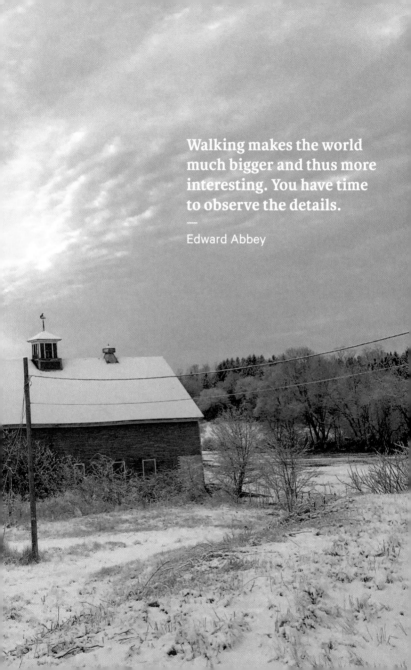

Walking makes the world much bigger and thus more interesting. You have time to observe the details.

—

Edward Abbey

Resources

Articles

An 'Awe Walk' Might Do Wonders for Your Well-Being
— Gretchen Reynolds, *New York Times*, 2020

Give Your Ideas Some Legs
— Marily Oppezzo and Daniel L. Schwartz, *Journal of Experimental Psychology*, 2014, apa.org

How Walking in Nature Changes the Brain
— Gretchen Reynolds, *New York Times*, 2015

One Foot in Front of the Other:
How a Daily Walk Helps Us Cope
— *New York Times*, 2020

Science's Newest Miracle Drug is Free
— Aaron Reuben, *Outside* magazine, 2019

Stepping Up Your Creativity
— *BrainWorld*, 2020

The Extraordinary Power of Going for a Walk
— Gloria Liu, *Outside* magazine, 2020

The Science of Why You Do Your Best Thinking While Walking
— Jessica Stillman, *Inc.* magazine

Walking and the Happy Brain
— Katie Arnold, *Outside* magazine, 2017

Walking as Creative Fuel
— Maria Popova, *Brain Pickings*

Walk Like a Buddha
— *Tricycle* magazine, 2011

Why Long Walks Will Change Your Life
— Harry J. Stead, *Human Parts*, 2020

Why Walking Helps Us Think
— Ferris Jabr, *The New Yorker*, 2014

Why We Walk
— Maria Popova, *Brain Pickings*

Books

In Praise of Walking — Shane O'Mara

Wanderlust — Rebecca Solnit

Podcasts

GirlTrek Uses Black Women's History to Encourage Walking
as a Healing Tradition
— *Morning Edition*, NPR, 2020

Why We Walk: The Bliss of Living One Step at a Time
— *On Point*, wbur, NPR

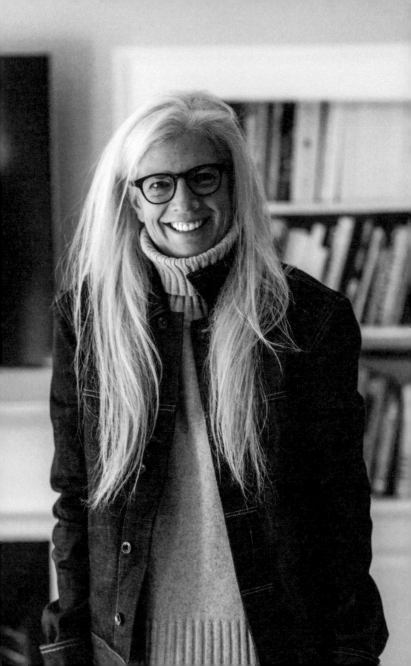

About the author

Libby DeLana is an award-winning executive creative director, designer/art director by trade, who has spent her career in the ad world. She was the Director of Design at MullenLowe for 15 years, then went on to co-found the agency Mechanica. Libby's work has been featured in *The One Show* awards (USA), *Cannes Lions*, and in publications including *D&AD*, *Fast Company*, *Graphis*, and *Communication Arts*. She has been profiled by the BBC Radio 4 series *The Chain* and several podcasts.

Libby is very committed to purpose-driven organisations and is currently on the Board of Directors for BlinkNow and The Jeanne Geiger Crisis Center and is an advisor to It's August, a brand reimagining and redefining the period experience.

She is an advocate for female leadership, an aspiring pilot, rookie fly fisher, fan of a strong cup of tea and mum to two tall, smart, kind men. *Do Walk* is her first published book.

You can connect with Libby on Instagram *@parkhere #thismorningwalk* and *libbydelana.com* or *thismorningwalk.com*

Thanks

Thanks to all my walking buddies:

Miranda, Claire, David, Orren, Will, Marta, Anna, Wanda, Hayley, Adam, Kourtney, Cheryl R, Faith, Gabriella, Gary, Charley, Patty, Cheryl S, Lauren, Karen, Maggie, Jeremy, Roda, Eric, Justin, Liz, Jen, Beth, Will, Nicole, Becky, Arabella, Kelsey, Kimberly, Becca, Eduardo, Steve L, Alfred, Elaine, Stephanie, Ellen, Cath, Wendy, Kai, Lacy, Amy, Janis, Ann, Paul, Eliza, Savannah, MaryJo, Syb, John, Sue, Tina, Patricia, Molly, Dominic, Marilyn, Gillian, John, Abbie, Lisa, Duke, Lee, Louisa, Dell, Zascha, Jessica, Alice, Kate, Charlotte

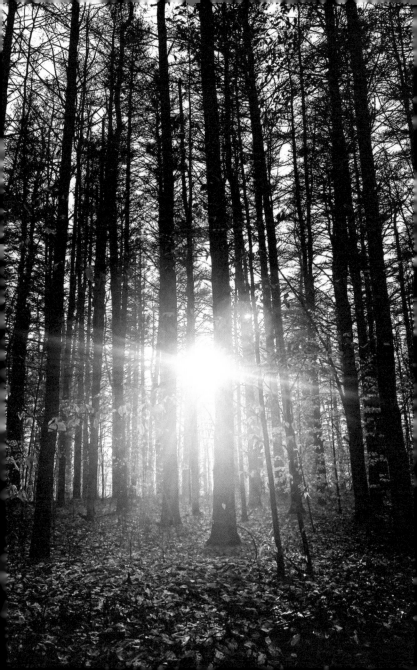

Books in the series

Do Agile Tim Drake

Do Beekeeping Orren Fox

Do Birth Caroline Flint

Do Breathe
    Michael Townsend Williams

Do Build Alan Moore

Do Death Amanda Blainey

Do Design Alan Moore

Do Disrupt Mark Shayler

Do Earth Tamsin Omond

Do Fly Gavin Strange

Do Grow Alice Holden

Do Improvise Robert Poynton

Do Inhabit Sue Fan, Danielle Quigley

Do Lead Les McKeown

Do Listen Bobette Buster

Do Make James Otter

Do Opportunity Steve Larosiliere

Do Open David Hieatt

Do Pause Robert Poynton

Do Photo Andrew Paynter

Do Present Mark Shayler

Do Preserve
    Anja Dunk, Jen Goss, Mimi Beaven

Do Protect Johnathan Rees

Do Purpose David Hieatt

Do Scale Les McKeown

Do Sea Salt
    Alison, David & Jess Lea-Wilson

Do Sing James Sills

Do Sourdough Andrew Whitley

Do Story Bobette Buster

Do Team Charlie Gladstone

Do Walk Libby DeLana

Do Wild Baking Tom Herbert

Also available

Path A short story about reciprocity Louisa Thomsen Brits

The Skimming Stone A short story about courage Dominic Wilcox

Stay Curious How we created a world class event in a cowshed Clare Hieatt

The Path of a Doer A simple tale of how to get things done David Hieatt

Available in print, digital and audio formats from booksellers or via our website: **thedobook.co**

To hear about events and forthcoming titles, you can find us on social media @dobookco, or subscribe to our newsletter